X #57 09

A Color Handbook

Small Animal Fluid, Electrolyte and Acid-base Disorders

Elisa Mazzaferro, MS, DVM, PhD, DACVECC

Cornell University Veterinary Specialists
Stamford, CT, USA

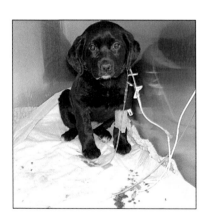

MANSON PUBLISHING

Copyright © 2013 Manson Publishing Ltd
ISBN: 978-1-84076-167-2

A CIP catalogue record for this book is available from the British Library.

For full details of all Manson Publishing Ltd titles please write to:
Manson Publishing Ltd, 73 Corringham Road, London NW11 7DL, UK.
Tel: +44(0)20 8905 5150
Fax: +44(0)20 8201 9233
Email: manson@mansonpublishing.com
Website: www.mansonpublishing.com

Commissioning editor: Jill Northcott
Project manager: Julie Bennett
Copy editor: Julie Pickard
Layout: DiacriTech, India
Colour reproduction: Tenon & Polert Colour Scanning Ltd, HK
Printed by: Butler Tanner and Dennis, Frome, UK

CONTENTS

PREFACE

Fluid therapy is one of the most important aspects of therapy in both small and large animal medicine. It is also extremely controversial, in that there are many opinions as to how to provide fluid therapy in different disease states. The descriptions provided within this text are meant to be used as guidelines that this author follows when implementing fluid and transfusion therapy. The text is divided into chapters that describe the physiologic fluid compartments within the body and how fluid travels from place to place within the body. The next chapter describes how to place and maintain intravenous and intraosseous catheters, as well as potential complications of intravenous catheterization. Next, the various types of crystalloid and colloid fluids and how they behave within the body are described. Transfusion medicine and electrolyte disorders are discussed in the next two chapters, followed by discussion of various forms of shock, resuscitation, and monitoring during shock states. The final chapter then describes clinical cases in which the concepts described in the text can be applied in daily practice. It is my hope that the readers will find this text useful when treating their own patients.

ABBREVIATIONS

ACD	acid–citrate–dextrose
ACT	activated clotting time
ACTH	adrenocorticotropic hormone
ADH	antidiuretic hormone
ADP	adenosine diphosphate
APTT	activated partial thromboplastin time
ATP	adenosine triphosphate
COP	colloid osmotic pressure
CPDA	citrate–phosphate–dextrose–adenine
CPP	cerebral perfusion pressure
CRI	constant-rate infusion
CRT	capillary refill time
CSF	cerebrospinal fluid
CVP	central venous pressure
D5W	5% dextrose in water
DEA	dog erythrocyte antigen
DIC	disseminated intravascular coagulation
DKA	diabetic ketoacidosis
DOCP	desoxycorticosterone pivalate
ECG	electrocardiogram
ELISA	enzyme-linked immunoabsorbent assay
FDP	fibrin degradation product
FeLV	feline leukemia virus
FFP	fresh frozen plasma
FIP	feline infectious peritonitis
FIV	feline immunodeficiency virus
FP	frozen plasma
GI	gastrointestinal
HBOC	hemoglobin-based oxygen carrier
ICP	intracranial pressure
IFA	immunofluorescent assay
MAP	mean arterial pressure
MODS	multiple organ dysfunction syndrome
PCR	polymerase chain reaction
PCV	packed cell volume
PN	parenteral nutrition
PPN	partial parenteral nutrition
pRBC	packed red blood cell
PT	prothrombin time
PTH	parathyroid hormone
REE	resting energy expenditure
RSAT	rapid slide agglutination test
SIADH	syndrome of inappropriate ADH secretion
SIRS	systemic inflammatory response syndrome
TAT	tube agglutination test
TBW	total body water
TPN	total parenteral nutrition
TS	total solids
VAP	vascular access port
VWf	von Willebrand factor

CHAPTER 1

Fluid compartments and total body water

- **Introduction**

- **Fluid compartments and total body water**

- **Fluid exchange between compartments**

- **Osmolality**

- **Dehydration versus hypovolemia**

- **Response to hypovolemia**

- **Maintenance fluid requirements**

- **Sensible and insensible fluid losses**

- **Fluid balance**

- **Measurement of 'ins and outs'**

- **Rehydration**

- **Conclusions**

INTRODUCTION

In small animal medicine, it is now considered to be the standard of care to administer intravenous fluids to any patient that has a condition that is associated with a lack of fluid intake or with fluid loss. Some persons may think that the science and thought processes behind fluid administration are mysterious and complex. However, fluid therapy can be simplified a little by first providing information about fluid composition and compartments within the body, describing how fluid moves from compartment to compartment, and how to recognize and treat fluid derangements, including hypovolemia and various degrees of dehydration.

FLUID COMPARTMENTS AND TOTAL BODY WATER

Water is essential for life. Without water, normal body functioning is impaired, and ultimately this can lead to death if therapeutic interventions are not implemented. A discussion of intravenous fluid administration would be incomplete without an understanding of total body water (TBW) and fluid balance between the various compartments within the body.

Water is a major contributor to an animal's body weight. An understanding of electrolyte and protein composition within the body is essential to help maintain homeostasis and to use the variety of fluids that are available to treat specific abnormalities. Approximately 60% of a healthy animal's total body weight is water. This value can change slightly depending on age, lean body mass, degree of leanness or obesity, and gender. For example, neonatal puppies and kittens have a relatively higher percentage of water in their bodies than adults. Adipose tissue contains more water than does muscle, and can contribute to a larger percentage of water in obese animals.

Water is located in separate yet intertwined compartments within the body. Conceptually, the body can be divided into the intracellular and extracellular compartments (**1**).

Intracellular fluid is located within cells, and contributes approximately two-thirds (66%) to total body water. Extracellular fluid is that which is located outside of cells, and contributes approximately one-third (33%) to total body water. Extracellular fluid can be further subdivided into the intravascular and interstitial compartments. The intravascular space contains fluid that is contained within blood vessels. It is through these vessels that plasma water, cellular components, proteins, and various electrolytes flow. The interstitial extravascular compartment is the space located outside of the blood vessels. Of this, intravascular fluid contributes only 8–10% of TBW, whereas interstitial fluid contributes 24% of TBW. A very small amount of fluid is known as transcellular fluid, and is located within the gastrointestinal tract, joints, cartilage, and cerebrospinal space.[1] It has been estimated that total body water is approximately 534–660 mL/kg in a healthy dog.[1] Total intravascular fluid volume has been estimated as 80–90 mL/kg in dogs and cats. Of that, the fluid component, or intravascular plasma water volume, has been estimated to be approximately 50 mL/kg in dogs, and 45 mL/kg in cats.[1]

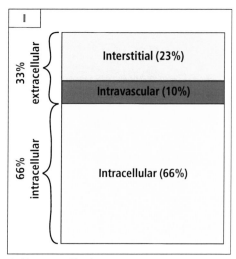

I Diagram of body water compartments.

FLUID EXCHANGE BETWEEN COMPARTMENTS

Total body water is in a constant state of flux between the various compartments within the body. The rate of fluid exchange largely depends on the forces that favor fluid retention within a compartment versus the forces that favor fluid movement or filtration from a compartment. The colloid osmotic pressure (COP) of a compartment is dictated by the concentration of protein within that space. Albumin is a protein which contributes approximately 80% to COP. Hydrostatic pressure is the pressure generated by the force of fluid within a compartment. The COP influences fluid retention within a compartment, while the hydrostatic pressure influences fluid movement from the compartment.

Starling's equation predicts fluid flux between compartments in the body (**2**).[2] The equation is as follows:

$$V = [kf(P_c - P_i) - \sigma(\pi_c - \pi_{if})] - Q_{lymph}$$

where kf = the filtration coefficient (varies from tissue to tissue within the body); P_c and P_i is the hydrostatic pressure within the capillary (P_c) and interstitial space (P_i), σ is the pore size of the capillary membrane and π describes the colloid effect of protein, such as albumin, in the capillary (π_c) and the interstitium (π_i). Finally, Q_{lymph} describes the rate of lymph flow from the interstitium.[2]

When hydrostatic forces exceed colloid osmotic forces, fluid will leave one compartment and go to the other (**2**). Conversely, a relative increase in colloid osmotic forces within a compartment can retain fluid within, or draw fluid into, the compartment. Flow of fluid from a compartment will increase the colloid osmotic pressure of that compartment, and then will increase the hydrostatic pressure of the compartment into which it moves. A more detailed explanation of a protein's effect on fluid flux within the body will be given in Chapter 4.

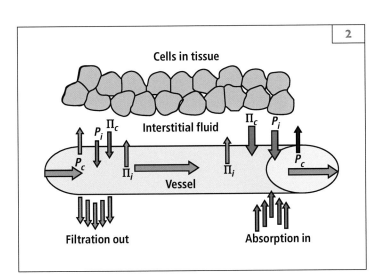

2 Diagram to illustrate Starling's equation of fluid flux between compartments in the body. P_c: hydrostatic pressure within the capillary; P_i: hydrostatic pressure within the interstitial space; π: the colloid effect of protein, such as albumin, in the capillary (π_c) and the interstitium (π_i).[2]

OSMOLALITY

The fluid compartments within the body hold various concentrations of small particles. Serum osmolality is determined by the number of osmotically active small particles in solution. Small particles can often readily diffuse through small pores in a capillary endothelium. The capillary endothelium is relatively impermeable to large particles such as proteins. This causes the larger particles to stay within the vascular and interstitial spaces, while the smaller particles are free to move across the vascular bed, depending on the concentration of the particles on either side of the vascular membrane. Any charged particle in solution can contribute to serum osmolality. The molecules that contribute the most to serum osmolality include sodium, potassium, chloride, bicarbonate, urea, and glucose.[1] Some particles, such as sodium, are transported across membranes with cotransport proteins, while others, such as urea, diffuse freely across the membrane from an area of greater concentration to an area of lower concentration until equilibrium is met. Normal serum osmolality is 290–310 mOsm/kg in dogs and cats. Serum osmolality can be calculated by the following formula:

$$\text{Osmolality (mOsm/liter)} = 2[(Na^+) + (K^+)] + [glucose]/18 + [BUN]/2.8^1$$

(NB. In the formula above, glucose and BUN are normally measured in mg/dL, rather than in mmol/L, so must be converted by the factors 18 and 2.8, respectively, for the units to be consistent.)

Osmolality can also be measured. In some cases, the presence of unmeasured solutes can increase the measured osmolality. The osmolal gap can be obtained by subtracting the calculated osmolality from the actual measured osmolality. Normally the osmolal gap is less than 10–15 mOsm/kg.

Hypotonic fluid loss, that is, the loss of fluid in excess of solute, can result in a relative increase in serum osmolality. Other conditions that can increase serum osmolality include Cushing's disease (hyperadrenocorticism), elevated serum aldosterone levels (which favors sodium retention), renal failure, diabetes insipidus, diabetes mellitus, and heat-induced illness (*Table 1*).[3] Osmoreceptors in the hypothalamus can sense moment to moment changes in serum osmolality. When osmolality increases due to increased intake of solutes or due to fluid loss in excess of solute, the hypothalamus triggers the release of antidiuretic hormone (ADH). ADH acts on the renal collecting ducts and opens water channels to favor water reabsorption and retention. Once the animal's osmolality has been normalized, the major contributors of serum osmolality are diluted, and ADH excretion from the hypothalamus ceases.

Table 1
Conditions that can increase serum osmolality and osmolal gap

Administration of:
Mannitol
Radiocontrast media
Sodium phosphate enemas
Diabetes mellitus
Elevations in serum:
Phosphate
Sodium
Sulfate
Ethylene glycol
Ethanol
Ketoacidosis (acetoacetate and/or β-hydroxybutyrate)
Lactic acidosis
Methanol
Parenteral nutrition
Renal failure
Salicylates
Salt intoxication

Isotonic fluid loss

Isotonic fluid loss is characterized by loss of fluid that has the same osmolality as plasma. For example, in a patient with a loss of renal concentrating ability and excessive urine loss, or a patient that is actively hemorrhaging, the fluid lost will not change serum osmolality. There will be no exchange of fluid from cells to alter interstitial or intravascular deficits. If isotonic fluid loss is excessive, the patient may exhibit clinical signs of hypovolemia.

Hypertonic fluid loss

Hypertonic fluid loss occurs when solutes are lost from the body. For example, in animals with sodium wasting, as seen in severe hypoadrenocorticism, the loss of solute, or sodium, can result in significant hyponatremia. Sodium is a major player that contributes to serum osmolality. The animal's serum osmolality will decrease and result in the shift of fluid into the interstitial and intracellular spaces, and this can result in cerebral edema. Too rapid correction of serum sodium by more than 15 mEq/L in a 24 hour period can potentially result in a condition called central pontine myelinolysis.[4]

DEHYDRATION VERSUS HYPOVOLEMIA

Dehydration refers to a decrease in TBW, whereas hypovolemia largely refers to inadequate circulating intravascular fluid volume. Dehydration can also be classified depending on the type of fluid lost, for example whether there is a pure water loss (loss of water without loss of solutes) or loss of water with solutes.[5]

Hypovolemia refers to inadequate circulating volume. Hypovolemia can result in hypovolemic shock from excessive hemorrhage, such as that observed with a bleeding splenic mass, vitamin K antagonist rodenticide intoxication, or arterial laceration. Hypovolemia can also occur due to severe fluid loss, and in end-stage dehydration, such as that observed in a puppy with parvoviral enteritis, or an elderly cat in end-stage renal failure. Parameters used to determine an animal's hydration status should not be used to determine its intravascular volume status (**3**). Intravascular fluid volume and cardiac output largely determine organ perfusion. In the peripheral tissues, measures of perfusion include capillary refill time (CRT) and mucous

3
PARAMETERS OF HYDRATION Skin turgor Sunken eyes Mucous membrane dryness Body weight
PARAMETERS OF PERFUSION Capillary refill time Mucous membrane color Arterial blood pressure Heart rate Urine output

3 Parameters of hydration versus parameters of perfusion.

membrane color. In the normal animal, the mucous membranes should be pink and moist, with a CRT of less than 2 seconds. Pale pink to whitish gray mucous membranes with a prolonged CRT can be found with either hypovolemic or cardiogenic shock. Other indirect markers of perfusion include urine output, blood pressure, and heart rate (*Table 2*).

Table 2
Estimations of dehydration and associated clinical signs (Adapted from Wingfield 2002)[6]

Estimated degree of dehydration	Clinical signs
< 5%	History of vomiting or diarrhea or other fluid loss, normal mucous membranes
5%	History of vomiting or diarrhea or other fluid loss, tacky or dry mucous membranes, mild skin tenting
7%	History of vomiting or diarrhea or other fluid loss, dry mucous membranes, increased skin tenting, tachycardia, normal pulse quality and arterial blood pressure
10%	History of vomiting or diarrhea or other fluid loss, dry mucous membranes, increased skin tenting, tachycardia, decreased pulse pressure
12%	History of vomiting or diarrhea or other fluid loss, dry mucous membranes, sunken eyes/dry cornea, increased skin tenting, tachy- or bradycardia, weak to absent pulses, hypotension, cold extremities, hypothermia, alteration of consciousness

RESPONSE TO HYPOVOLEMIA

Baroreceptors are located in the carotid body and aortic arch which sense the stretch of the vessel walls, depending on how much intravascular circulating fluid is present. In healthy, euvolemic animals, stimulation of the stretch receptors triggers the vagus nerve to slow the heart rate. When there is a decrease in circulating intravascular fluid volume, the stretch receptors sense a decrease in wall tension and reduced firing of vagal stimuli to the brain. This allows the sympathetic nervous system to manifest itself and results in a reflex increase in heart rate in an attempt to maintain cardiac output in the face of decreased intravascular fluid volume (**4**). In the early stage of hypovolemic shock, the heart rate and blood pressure may be normal if compensation is adequate, or there may be tachycardia with hypotension as compensatory mechanisms can no longer maintain cardiac output. As hypovolemia progresses, the sympathetic output can become exhausted and no longer allows an increase in cardiac output and blood pressure. As a result, heart rate and cardiac contractility decrease. Sympathetic tone of the vasculature is decreased and vessels dilate as a result. In late decompensatory shock, perfusion parameters worsen markedly and are manifested as bradycardia, prolonged CRT, hypotension, pale pink to whitish gray or cyanotic mucous membranes, decreased central venous pressure, and decreased urine output (*Table 3*). In this clinical situation, rapid and aggressive intravenous fluid resuscitation is necessary to save the animal's life.

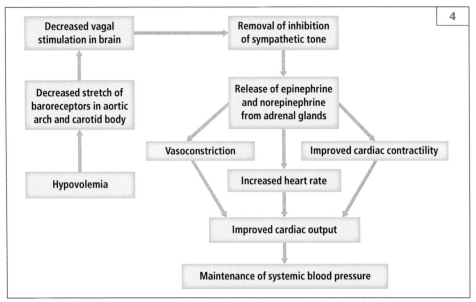

4 Diagram of baroreceptor-mediated feedback during early hypovolemic shock. Efforts to maintain cardiac output and systemic arterial blood pressure in the face of decreased circulating intravascular fluid volume. (After Day TK, Bateman S [2006]. Shock syndromes. In: DiBartola SP (ed). *Fluid, Electrolyte, and Acid–Base Disorders in Small Animal Practice*, 3rd edn. Saunders Elsevier, St Louis, p. 542.)

Table 3
Stages of shock and associated clinical signs

Stage of shock	Clinical signs	
Compensatory	Tachycardia	Normal to rapid CRT
	Hyperemic or normal color	Normotensive
	to mucous membranes	Normothermic
Early decompensatory	Tachycardia	
	Normal to pale mucous membranes	
	Rapid CRT	
	Normo- to slightly hypotensive	
	Normo- to hypothermic	
Late decompensatory	Bradycardia	Pale mucous membranes
	Delayed CRT	Hypotensive
	Hypothermic	

MAINTENANCE FLUID REQUIREMENTS

An animal's maintenance fluid requirements are based on its lean body mass. In the past, there have been numerous estimates of maintenance fluid requirements for dogs and cats. The recommendations have largely been extrapolated from data obtained in human studies, or from experiments in research animals. In recent years, data have been obtained in healthy dogs and dogs with critical illness to determine the animal's daily caloric requirement, the resting energy expenditure (REE). Although it may seem inappropriate to discuss REE in a fluid therapy text, it is actually necessary when considering an animal's metabolic water requirements. To metabolize one kilocalorie of energy, 1 mL of water is consumed. Therefore, calculation of an animal's REE can be extrapolated to determine the volume of fluid required in a 24 hour period for metabolic purposes.[7]

A linear equation to calculate an animal's REE and metabolic water requirements is as follows:

$$REE^* = mL\ H_2O^* = [(30 \times body\ weight\ in\ kg)] + 70$$

* denotes requirement for a 24 hour period

This formula is accurate for animals weighing more than 2 kg and less than 100 kg (**5**). An important thing to remember is that

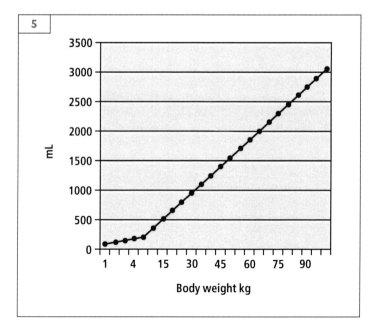

5 Daily fluid requirements are based on an animal's metabolism. Previous suggestions for administration of intravenous fluid tended to underhydrate animals of lower body weight, and overhydrate animals at the larger end of the spectrum. Metabolic water requirements are based on the formula (30 × body weight in kilograms) + 70 = mL water/day.

the REE is obtained in a healthy, euvolemic animal, who is resting and in a post-prandial state. This is often not the case in a dehydrated or hypovolemic animal in clinical practice, but is a place from where to start. Many patients have excessive fluid loss in the form of diarrhea, vomitus, decreased renal concentrating ability, and are stressed, so are not eating. Careful weighing of the animal on a regular basis allows the clinician to determine whether interstitial and intracellular dehydration is being corrected, by matching fluid input with the animal's ongoing losses (*Table 4*).

Table 4
Daily maintenance fluid requirements based on body weight

kg Body weight	mL Water per day	Approximate mL/hr
1	100	4
2	130	5
3	160	7
4	190	8
5	220	9
10	370	15
15	520	21
20	670	28
25	820	34
30	970	40
35	1120	47
40	1270	53
45	1420	60
50	1570	65
55	1720	71
60	1870	78
65	2020	84
70	2170	90
75	2320	97
80	2470	103
85	2620	109
90	2770	115
95	2920	122
100	3070	128

SENSIBLE AND INSENSIBLE FLUID LOSSES

Sensible fluid losses are those that can be measured, and include fluid lost in the form of urine, feces, vomitus, and wound exudates (6). Accurate quantitation of urine output should be performed by collecting the urine as a free-catch sample, or in a closed collection system attached to a urinary catheter. In cases where this is not possible, weighing the bedding of the animal before and after urination, vomiting, or diarrhea on the bedding can allow the clinician to estimate fluid loss. In such cases, 1 g is approximately equivalent to 1 mL of water. Similarly, weighing an animal's bandage material prior to placement can allow the clinician to calculate the amount of fluid loss in the form of wound exudates.

Insensible losses are those which cannot be measured, and include sweat, saliva, and excessive panting. Normally, insensible losses are estimated to be 20–30 mL/kg/day.

FLUID BALANCE

Fluid balance in healthy animals is a function of the fluid that is taken in or created during metabolic processes versus the fluid that is lost in urine, feces, vomitus, and respiration. Fluid is normally ingested in the form of water or within foodstuffs. Canned soft food products contain more water on a dry matter basis than hard dry kibble. Fluid loss varies between individual patients, but under normal circumstances is balanced with intake such that in a healthy animal total body water remains essentially the same. Excessive loss of fluid can occur during conditions with hemorrhage, vomiting, diarrhea, burn and wound exudates, and excessive panting (7). Rapid changes in body weight on an hour-to-hour basis are largely due to changes in total body water. Knowledge of an animal's weight and estimates of hydration and dehydration parameters can be extrapolated to determine fluid deficits during states of illness, and to aid in the calculation of fluid requirements during states of health and diseases that are associated with fluid loss (*Table 5*).

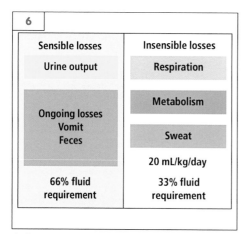

6	
Sensible losses	**Insensible losses**
Urine output	**Respiration**
	Metabolism
Ongoing losses **Vomit** **Feces**	**Sweat**
	20 mL/kg/day
66% fluid requirement	**33% fluid requirement**

6 Sensible and insensible fluid losses. Sensible losses can be measured; insensible losses must be estimated and total 20–30 mL/kg/day. The sum of sensible and insensible losses equals the term 'outs' when measuring 'ins' and 'outs' for a patient.

7 For this patient with severe thrombocytopenia the vomitus is excessive, and also contains digested blood.

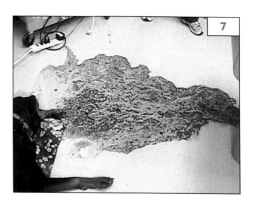

Table 5
Fluid administration requirements (mL/hour) to administer maintenance fluids plus correction of varying degrees of dehydration over a 24 hour period

kg Body weight	5% Dehydration	7% Dehydration	10% Dehydration	12% Dehydration
1	6	7	8	9
2	9	11	13	15
3	13	16	20	22
4	16	20	25	28
5	19	24	30	34
10	36	44	57	65
15	52	59	84	96
20	70	86	76	128
25	86	107	138	159
30	103	128	165	190
35	120	149	193	222
40	136	170	220	253
45	154	191	248	285
50	169	211	273	315
55	186	231	300	346
60	203	253	328	378
65	219	274	355	409
70	236	213	381	440
75	253	318	410	472
80	270	336	436	503
85	286	248	463	534
90	303	378	490	565
95	320	399	518	597
100	336	420	545	628

MEASUREMENTS OF 'INS AND OUTS'

In some critically ill animals fluid losses can exceed fluid intake, and can lead to dehydration despite the administration of intravenous or enteral fluids. In other animals with marginal renal function, fluid intake can exceed fluid output and can lead to intravascular and interstitial volume overload. Both scenarios can ultimately increase patient morbidity and mortality.

The practice of 'ins and outs' requires calculation of fluid being infused into the animal compared with sensible and insensible fluid losses (8). In a rehydrated, euvolemic patient 'ins' should ideally equal 'outs' in order to maintain hydration and intravascular volume status without causing fluid overload.

8

INS: What has the animal received over the past 6 hr?
$$45 \text{ mL/hr} \quad 6 \text{ hr} = 270 \text{ mL}$$

OUTS: Outs can be subdivided into sensible and insensible losses.

Sensible losses:
Vomitus	60 g = approximately 60 mL
Diarrheic feces	90 g = approximately 90 mL
Urine	100 g = approximately 100 mL

Insensible losses = 20–30 mL/kg/day
Conservatively, 20 mL/kg/day   10 kg = 200 mL/day   24 hr = 8.3 mL/hr
8.3 mL/hr   6 hr = 50 mL

Total losses:
60 mL vomitus + 90 mL diarrhea + 100 mL urine + 50 mL insensible = 300 mL

'INS'	vs.	'OUTS'
270 mL		300 mL

Take-home message: For this patient, if the fluid losses continue the animal will be in a constant state of fluid deficit. The amount of intravenous fluids that the animal is receiving must be increased. One way to do this is to replace the fluid deficit (in this case, 30 mL) over the next 6 hour period, in addition to the original rate of fluid administration (45 mL/hr). In this case, the intravenous fluid rate could be increased by 5 mL/hr (to 50 mL/hr), and reassessed (recalculated) after 6 hours. Any ongoing losses should continue to be weighed, as well as the animal, to make sure the patient's fluid deficit and ongoing losses are matched by intake.

---

8 Calculation of 'ins and outs' over 6 hours for a 10 kg animal who has vomited a measured amount of 60 g of vomitus, has defecated 90 g of diarrhea, and has produced a total of 100 mL of urine. At the time of initial presentation the animal was estimated to be 7% dehydrated, but the fluid deficit has been replaced over the past 36 hours. The patient is currently on 45 mL/hr of a balanced crystalloid intravenous fluid solution.

REHYDRATION

Once a clinician subjectively determines an animal's degree of dehydration, the volume of fluid that must be administered to replace the fluid deficit can be calculated by the following formula:

% dehydration × body weight in kg × 1000
= mL fluid deficit

The fluid deficit then should be added to the animal's maintenance fluid requirements. Controversy exists on how fast an animal's fluid deficit must be replaced. Some clinicians replace the deficit over 4–6 hours, while others choose to replace 80–100 % of the deficit over 24 hours. There is no absolute correct or incorrect method of replacing an animal's fluid deficit, as long as the deficit is considered in the calculation of the total amount of fluids that need to be administered to a dehydrated patient. So, for example, a 30 kg dog presents with a 24 hour history of vomiting and diarrhea after ingesting garbage. The dog's mucous membranes are dry, and there is increased skin tenting. The dog's heart rate is 150 beats per minute, and the femoral pulses are of good quality and synchronous with the heartbeat. How much fluid should be administered to replace his dehydration? Remember to include his maintenance requirements, too!

Given the parameters of increased skin tenting, dry mucous membranes, tachycardia and good femoral pulse quality, it is estimated that the dog is subjectively 7% dehydrated. Therefore,

$0.07 \times 30 \text{ kg} \times 1000 = 2100 \text{ mL fluid deficit}$

Maintenance: $(30 \times 30) + 70 = 970 \text{ mL}$

Adding the two together: $(2100 + 970) = 3070$ mL to be administered over the next 24 hours, plus any additional ongoing losses that might occur if the patient continues to have vomiting and diarrhea. See, that wasn't that difficult, was it?

CONCLUSIONS

The administration of intravenous fluids requires an understanding of the type of fluid lost, the presence of underlying disease processes, the animal's hydration and intravascular volume status, the animal's ability to retain fluid within the vasculature, and determinants of resuscitation end-points when treating dehydration and various forms of shock. When the fluid deficits in the interstitial and intracellular spaces are replenished, clinical signs associated with dehydration (i.e. increased skin turgor, dry mucous membranes, sunken eyes) will resolve. Similarly, when the intravascular fluid volume is replenished during states of hypovolemia, heart rate, blood pressure, CRT, and urine output will normalize. Types of crystalloid and colloid solutions, indications on how to administer fluids, potential complications of fluid therapy, and fluid therapy for specific disease states will be discussed in later chapters.

CHAPTER 2

Techniques and complications of vascular access

- **Introduction**

- **Types of intravenous catheters**

- **Peripheral venous catheters**

- **Central venous catheters**

- **Intraosseous catheterization**

- **Arterial catheterization**

- **Vascular cutdown**

- **The three-syringe blood sampling technique**

- **Maintenance of the intravenous catheter**

- **Complications associated with intravenous catheterization**

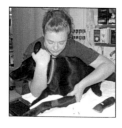 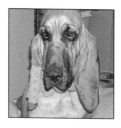 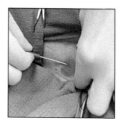 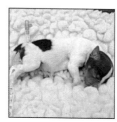

INTRODUCTION

Careful intravenous fluid administration is one of the most important aspects of care of the emergent patient. The placement of an intravenous catheter for the administration of intravenous fluids is important in the correction of acid–base and electrolyte abnormalities, to replace intravascular and interstitial fluid volume deficits, and to treat or prevent dehydration or hypovolemic shock. Vascular access is also important for the administration of drugs, blood products, and parenteral nutrition. For these reasons, the placement and maintenance of intravenous catheters are among the most important techniques to master in any veterinary hospital. Blood samples can be collected from larger bore catheters to prevent the need for uncomfortable repeated venipuncture. The benefits of vascular access are undoubtedly numerous, but are not altogether innocuous, and in some cases can result in complications that can contribute to patient morbidity. Care must therefore be taken to avoid inherent risks associated with intravenous catheterization. In the rare event that an intravenous catheter cannot be placed due to peripheral edema, extreme dehydration or hypotension, thrombophlebitis, generalized skin lesions, or coagulopathies, surgical cutdown to a vessel or placement of an intraosseous catheter may be necessary.

TYPES OF INTRAVENOUS CATHETERS

Intravenous catheters can be classified according to catheter type or location of placement. Peripheral venous catheters are placed in peripheral vessels, whereas central venous catheters are either placed in a central vessel such as the jugular vein, or inserted in a peripheral vessel with the distal tip of the catheter located in a central vein such as the caudal vena cava. Usually, peripheral catheters are shorter catheters that are used primarily for administration of colloid and crystalloid fluids, drugs, and blood products. Depending on the diameter of the catheter, blood may or may not be able to be withdrawn from the catheter, making venipuncture necessary at times for collection of blood samples.

Central venous catheters come in a variety of diameters and lengths, depending on their intended use and size of the patient (*Table 6*). Central venous catheters are often larger gauge than peripheral catheters, and longer, in order to sit in a central vein. Larger bore longer catheters are necessary for administration of hypertonic solutions that may cause thrombophlebitis in a smaller vessel. In addition to administration of colloid and crystalloid fluids and blood products, central venous catheters are also often used for blood sample collection and intravascular fluid volume monitoring by measuring central venous pressures (*Table 7* see p. 24).[1]

Table 6
French *vs*. gauge labeling of catheters

Single-lumen catheters are labeled by catheter gauge, and multi-lumen catheters are labeled by French size, both of which refer to the outer diameter of the catheter. Within a multi-lumen catheter the individual catheters themselves are described by catheter gauge.

French	Inches	Gauge
	0.016	27
	0.018	26
	0.020	25
	0.022	24
	0.024	23
	0.028	22
	0.032	21
	0.035	20
3	0.039	
	0.042	19
	0.049	18
4	0.053	
	0.058	17
	0.065	16
5	0.066	
	0.072	15
6	0.079	
7	0.092	
	0.083	14
	0.095	13
8	0.105	
	0.109	12
9	0.118	
	0.120	11
10	0.131	
	0.134	10
11	0.144	
12	0.158	
13	0.170	
14	0.184	
15	0.197	
16	0.210	

Table 7
Types, locations, indications, and contraindications of various intravenous catheters

Catheter type	Location	Indications	Contraindications
Short peripheral catheter	Cephalic	Fluid therapy, drug and blood product administration; used in animals with urinary or fecal incontinence or diarrhea	Thrombophlebitis or skin injury or infection over cephalic vein; avoid in animals who are vomiting, or have ptyalism, seizures, or epistaxis
	Lateral saphenous	Fluid therapy, drug and blood product administration; used in animals with vomiting, or who have ptyalism, seizures or epistaxis	Thrombophlebitis or skin injury or infection over lateral saphenous vein; avoid in animals who are incontinent or have diarrhea
	Medial saphenous	Fluid therapy, drug and blood product administration; used in animals with vomiting, or who have ptyalism, seizures or epistaxis	Thrombophlebitis or skin injury or infection over medial saphenous vein; avoid in animals who are incontinent or have diarrhea
Long single-lumen central catheter	Jugular	Fluid therapy, drug and blood product administration, repeated blood sample collection, parenteral nutrition; used in animals with urinary or fecal incontinence or diarrhea	Coagulopathies, hypercoagulable state; avoid in animals with increased intracranial pressure, seizures, or thrombophlebitis or skin injury or infection over jugular vein

Catheter type	Location	Indications	Contraindications
	Lateral saphenous	Fluid therapy, drug and blood product administration, repeated blood sample collection, parenteral nutrition; used in animals with vomiting, or who have ptyalism, seizures or epistaxis	Avoid in animals with thrombophlebitis or skin injury or infection over lateral saphenous vein, avoid in animals who are incontinent or have diarrhea
	Medial saphenous	Fluid therapy, drug and blood product administration, repeated blood sample collection, parenteral nutrition; used in animals with vomiting, or who have ptyalism, seizuresor epistaxis	Avoid in animals with thrombophlebitis or skin injury or infection over medial saphenous vein, avoid in animals who are incontinent or have diarrhea
Long multi-lumen central catheter	Jugular	Fluid therapy, drug and blood product administration, repeated blood sample collection, parenteral nutrition; used in animals with urinary or fecal incontinence or diarrhea	Coagulopathies, hypercoagulable state; avoid in animals with increased intracranial pressure, seizures, or thrombophlebitis or skin injury or infection over jugular vein
	Lateral saphenous	Fluid therapy, drug and blood product administration, repeated blood sample collection, parenteral nutrition; used in animals with vomiting, or who have ptyalism, seizures or epistaxis	Avoid in animals with thrombophlebitis or skin injury or infection over lateral saphenous vein, avoid in animals who are incontinent or have diarrhea

(*Continued*)

Table 7
Types, locations, indications, and contraindications of various intravenous catheters (*Continued*)

Catheter type	Location	Indications	Contraindications
	Medial saphenous	Fluid therapy, drug and blood product administration, repeated blood sample collection, parenteral nutrition; used in animals with vomiting, or who have ptyalism, seizures or epistaxis	Avoid in animals with thrombophlebitis or skin injury or infection over medial saphenous vein, avoid in animals who are incontinent or have diarrhea
Intraosseous	Intraosseous	Fluid therapy, drug and blood product administration; used when intravenous catheter placement is impossible due to patient size, hypovolemia, hypothermia, hypotension	Avoid if infection or injury over site of catheter placement; can be painful

PERIPHERAL VENOUS CATHETERS

Placement of a peripheral catheter is similar for cephalic, lateral saphenous, and medial saphenous veins. In general, the cephalic vein is the most commonly used site for catheter placement due to ease of placement and patient restraint.[2] However, in animals with very short limbs, cephalic catheter placement may be problematic when the animal pulls its leg towards the body, as the catheter can become occluded at the crook of the elbow. Also in patients that are vomiting, salivating, or having seizures, placement of a catheter at this site is relatively contraindicated due to the potential for catheter contamination or danger to personnel during a seizure. Instead, the lateral or medial saphenous veins may be more appropriate under these circumstances. Catheter placement in the hindlimbs is relatively contraindicated in patients with diarrhea or urinary or fecal incontinence, as contamination of the catheter site can occur.

The supplies necessary for a peripheral catheter include a clipper with clean blades, antimicrobial scrub and sterile saline or antimicrobial solution, gauze squares, 1 inch (12 mm) adhesive medical tape, the catheter, heparinized flush solution, and either a t-port or a male adapter to place in the catheter hub (**9**).

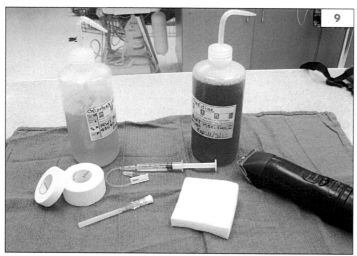

9 Supplies needed for placement of an intravenous catheter include clean clipper and blades, antimicrobial scrub solution, sterile gauze, intravenous catheter of choice, 0.5 inch (12 mm) and 1 inch (24 mm) white surgical tape, heparinized saline flush, and either a t-port or a male adapter.

The proper restraints for placement of cephalic, lateral saphenous, and medial saphenous catheters are displayed in Figures 10–12, respectively.

To place a peripheral intravenous catheter, the fur is clipped circumferentially around the patient's limb, taking care to clip long fur so that the fur does not contaminate the site of catheter entrance. An assistant then occludes the vessel, proximal to the site of catheter placement, such that the vessel becomes engorged and more visible or palpable (13). Visualization and/or palpation of the vessel may be difficult in animals that are obese, severely dehydrated, hypovolemic, hypotensive, or hypothermic. Next, the catheter is held at an approximately 30° angle, and pushed through the skin into the vessel (14). The skin can sometimes be very

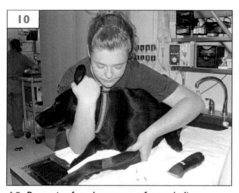

10 Restraint for placement of a cephalic intravenous catheter involves holding the patient's head close to the handler's body, to prevent movement and potential danger of biting. The handler holds the forelimb forward by pushing the elbow, and simultaneously occludes drainage from the cephalic vein by pushing at the dorsal (anterior) portion of the patient's elbow.

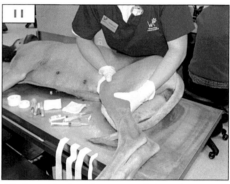

11 Restraint for placement of a lateral saphenous catheter involves placing the patient in lateral recumbency, and having an assistant place their forearm over/across the patient's neck, to prevent the patient from rising. With their other hand, the assistant holds the rear limb and occludes drainage from the lateral saphenous vein by placing pressure at the caudal aspect of the hindlimb, just proximal to the tarsus, distal to the stifle.

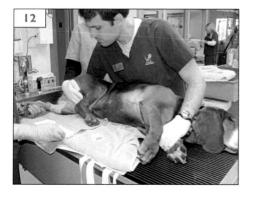

12 Restraint for placement of a medial saphenous catheter involves placing the patient in lateral recumbency, and holding the head with one hand to prevent the patient moving or biting the operator. With their other hand, the assistant bends the hindlimb on top towards the patient's ventral abdomen, and with the edge of their hand occludes outflow from the medial saphenous vein proximal to the stifle, in the inguinal region.

tough in intact male cats, or patients with significant dehydration. To prevent burring of the catheter tip as it enters the skin, it is sometimes necessary to perform percutaneous facilitation. Percutaneous facilitation refers to a technique in which the sharp bevel of an 18 or 20 gauge needle is used to make a nick incision gently in the skin over the vessel. This technique has also been called 'facilitative incision' or 'relief hole' (**15**).[2] When performing this technique, care must be taken to avoid lacerating the underlying vessel. The catheter is then placed through the nick incision in the skin, into the vessel.

After the catheter is placed through the skin, either with or without percutaneous facilitation, a flash of blood should be seen in the hub of the stylette (**16**).

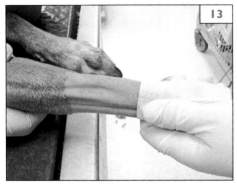

13 Close-up image of assistant occluding outflow from a dog's cephalic vein by placing pressure on the anterior portion of the limb, just distal or at the crook of the elbow.

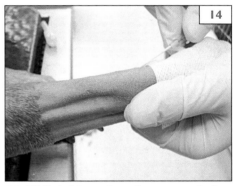

14 While holding a piece of gauze over the fur on the distal extremity, the operator prepares to insert a catheter into the patient's cephalic vein by holding the catheter at a 15–30° angle over the vein.

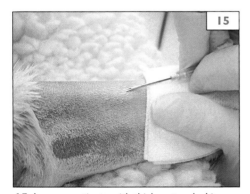

15 In some patients with thick or tough skin, it may be necessary to make a nick through the skin over the vessel. This can be accomplished with the sharp bevel of a hypodermic needle. This technique is known as 'percutaneous facilitation'.

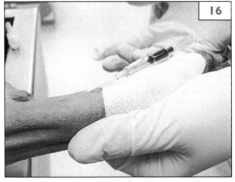

16 Once the catheter and stylette is in the vessel, blood will flow into the catheter hub.

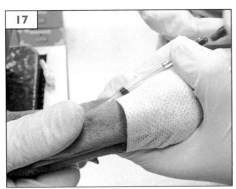

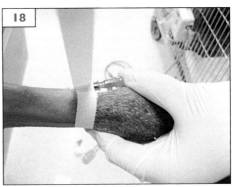

17 Once a flash of blood has been observed in the catheter hub, the catheter and its stylette should be advancved another 1–2 mm, then the catheter is pushed off the stylette, into the vessel. The assistant, with gloved hands, places pressure with a finger just proximal to the catheter entrance site, to prevent blood flow from the catheter hub during removal of the stylette and placement of a t-port or male adapter plug.

18 A piece of 0.5 inch (12 mm) white surgical adhesive tape is placed around the clean, dry catheter hub and around the limb. If the catheter hub is not secured within this initial piece of tape, the entire catheter can easily fall out of the vessel.

Once the flash of blood is observed, the catheter and stylette are advanced another 1–2 mm into the vessel, and the catheter is pushed off the stylette, into the vessel. Once the catheter is seated in the vessel, the person restraining the animal can gently occlude the vessel just proximal to the site of catheter insertion, to prevent blood from leaking from the catheter hub. The assistant should be wearing gloves, to prevent contamination of the catheter site (**17**). The flushed t-port or male adapter is then inserted, and the catheter is taped in place.[2]

To tape the catheter in place, the catheter hub and surrounding skin must be pristine and dry, to allow the tape to adhere securely to the skin. If the catheter hub or skin is wet or contaminated with blood, the adhesive on the tape will not stick and the catheter will spin inside the tape, and often dislodge from the vessel and fall out.

First, a strip of 0.5 inch (12 mm) white adhesive surgical tape is placed around the catheter hub (**18**) and wrapped securely around the limb. A length of 1 inch (24 mm) white adhesive surgical tape is then placed under the catheter hub and around the limb (**19**). Finally, a third length of tape is secured over the catheter hub, and around the limb. If a t-port is used, a fourth piece of tape can be secured around the t-port, then secured around the limb (**20**), taking care to avoid kinking the t-port tubing, as a kink in the t-port tubing will occlude the flow of fluid into the catheter.

Placement and taping of a lateral saphenous catheter is identical to that for a cephalic catheter. For lateral or medial saphenous vein catheterization, the patient is placed in lateral recumbency (**21**). Medial saphenous catheters are often placed in cats and small dogs with short limbs, such as Dachshunds and brachycephalic breeds such as Pekingese, Shih Tzu, and Pugs.[2] The medial saphenous vein can often be visualized between the inguinal area and the stifle (**22**). Taping the medial saphenous catheter in place follows the same protocol as taping other catheters, with the exception of securing the end of the t-port on the lateral aspect of the limb to allow easier access to the catheter.

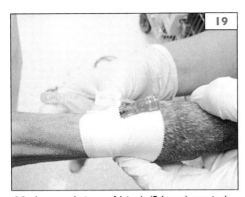

19 A second piece of 1 inch (24 mm) surgical adhesive tape is placed under the catheter hub, around the limb, then over the catheter hub to further secure the catheter in place within the vessel.

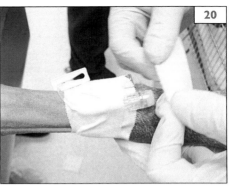

20 A third piece of surgical adhesive tape is placed under the catheter hub and t-port, then around the limb and over the top of the t-port to further secure the catheter in place.

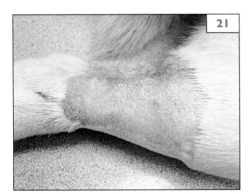

21 Location of the medial saphenous vein as it courses in between the stifle and hock, on the medial aspect of the limb. This photo demonstrates that the patient's skin is sensitive and can easily be abraded by clipper blades. Care should be exercised to avoid any abrasions or lacerations that can predispose the animal to catheter-related infection.

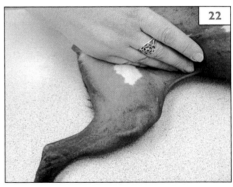

22 The medial saphenous vein can often be visualized between the inguinal area and the stifle.

Auricular catheter

In some breeds with large ears and auricular veins, such as Dachshunds and hound breeds, intravenous catheters can be placed in the ears (**23**).[2] The dorsolateral aspect of the ear surface is clipped, and aseptically prepared as described previously. Several gauze 4 × 4 inch (100 mm × 100 mm) squares are rolled and secured with 1 inch (25 mm) adhesive tape. The gauze roll is placed under the ear and the ear is molded over the gauze roll. The auricular vein should be visible on the dorsolateral aspect of the pinna. The ear is held flat over the clinician's fingers, and the vessel occluded proximally in between the index and middle fingers. The catheter is inserted through the skin directly into the vessel by holding the catheter parallel to the ear (**24**). Once a flash of blood is observed, the catheter is advanced into the vessel and secured in place with lengths of tape around the ear. Gauze rolls are used to stabilize the ear and prevent the catheter from becoming dislodged or kinking (**25**). Auricular catheters are often used during surgery and in extremely critical patients. Once an animal is mobile, placement of a different peripheral or central catheter often becomes necessary as auricular catheters are easily dislodged with patient movement.

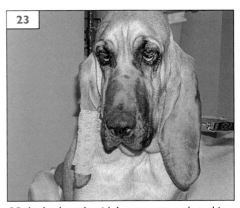

23 In dog breeds with longer ears, such as this Bloodhound, catheter can be placed in the auricular veins.

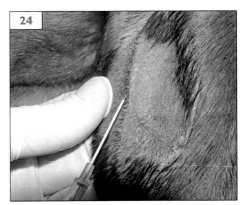

24 The dorsal, lateral aspect of the patient's ear is clipped and aseptically prepared. By holding the ear flat, and simultaneously occluding outflow of blood from the auricular vein, the operator can insert a catheter on the dorsal aspect of the ear.

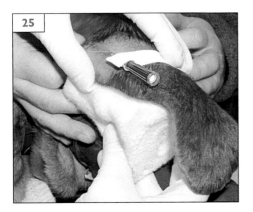

25 Following insertion of the catheter into the auricular vein, a piece of 0.5 inch (12 mm) surgical adhesive tape is placed around the catheter hub. To secure the catheter in place, prevent movement, and make the tape easier to secure around the ear, pieces of rolled up gauze are placed on the ventral surface of the ear, and the tape is then placed around the bundle.

CENTRAL VENOUS CATHETERS

Central venous catheters are longer catheters whose tip terminates in the cranial or caudal vena cava, just outside the heart.[1] In most cases, these catheters are placed in the external jugular vein, or the lateral or medial saphenous veins. In some patients, the catheter can be placed in a cephalic vein and run through the azygous vein to the cranial vena cava. In general, central venous catheters tend to be longer and larger in diameter than peripherally placed catheters, and are used for frequent blood sample collection or the administration of hypertonic solutions such as in parenteral nutrition.[1]

Through-the-needle catheters

Through-the-needle catheters are available in many lengths for placement into a central vein. Long catheters can be placed into the jugular, medial and lateral saphenous veins, and into cephalic veins in larger dogs. In most cases, the patient is too ill to require sedation, but should receive appropriate analgesia as warranted. Some patients who are more mobile and active may require light sedation for placement of a central venous catheter.

Over-the-wire catheters (Seldinger technique)

Over-the-wire catheter placement is also known as the Seldinger technique. Over-the-wire catheters are available in a variety of lengths and diameters. Some are available as single-lumen catheters, and others are available as multi-lumen catheters, which have multiple infusion ports at the proximal end that attach to individual catheters within the catheter lumen. Once the various components of the over-the-wire kit become familiar, this catheterization technique is actually very simple, and allows the placement of a long-lasting catheter with multiple uses.

The components of the over-the-wire catheter are generally similar from different manufacturers. Most kits contain both over-the-needle short intravenous catheters and similar gauge hypodermic needles, a vascular dilator, a J-wire, and the long catheter (**26**).

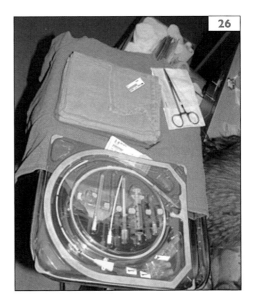

26 Example of a prefabricated kit for an over-the-wire catheter. Most kits include an over-the-needle catheter and/or hypodermic needle, J-wire and J-wire introducer, vascular dilator, and over-the-wire catheter.

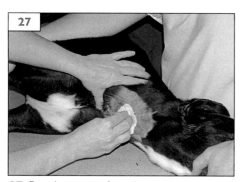

27 For placement of a catheter into the jugular vein, the patient is placed in lateral recumbency and the lateral neck clipped from the ramus of the mandible to the thoracic inlet.

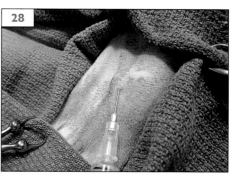

28 After aseptically preparing the area over the vessel, the skin is tented and the area over the vessel is infiltrated with a small amount of local anesthetic, such as 0.5–1 mg/kg lidocaine.

Some kits may also contain a syringe, ampoule of local anesthetic, antimicrobial wipes, sterile field towels, a scalpel blade, and male adapters. Although the extra components are convenient, they often add expense to the catheter kit, and may be acquired more economically from the hospital stock. Other supplies that are required for placement of an over-the-wire catheter include sterile gloves, clippers with clean blades, antimicrobial scrub and solution, nonabsorbable suture, thumb forceps, needle holder, sterile drapes or field towels, and a bandage kit.

Over-the-wire catheters can be placed in the jugular, medial saphenous, and lateral saphenous veins.[1] To place a jugular catheter, the patient is positioned in lateral recumbency, and the lateral aspect of the neck is clipped, from the ramus of the mandible to the thoracic inlet, and dorsally and ventrally to the midline of the neck (**27**) taking care to clip long fur that can potentially contaminate the catheter entrance site. The lateral neck is then aseptically scrubbed, allowing adequate contact time. The scrub is then rinsed off the skin with sterile saline, sterile water, or antimicrobial solution. Once the catheter site is properly clipped,

cleaned, and draped with sterile towels, a small amount of local anesthetic is injected into the skin over the proposed site of catheter insertion (**28**). Care must be taken to avoid injecting the local anesthetic directly into the vessel. Once the local anesthetic has taken effect, the skin is tented and a very small nick incision is made in the site using a number 11 scalpel blade (**29**), carefully avoiding lacerating the underlying vessel. Either an over-the-needle catheter or a hypodermic needle is then inserted through the nick incision in the skin into the vessel, similar to placing a short catheter into the same vessel (**30**). Once a flash of blood is observed in the catheter hub, the stylette is removed. Blood should flow freely from the hub of the catheter (**31**).

The next step is to insert the J-wire through the catheter or needle hub, into the vessel (**32**). The J-wire is usually seated in an adapter that will fit securely in the catheter or needle hub. The J-wire can be pulled back into the adapter initially, then once the wire is pushed into the vessel, the flexible wire opens up into the characteristic J shape, which prevents it from penetrating the wall of the vessel or heart (**33**).

29 The skin is tented and a nick incision is made over the vessel, taking care to avoid lacerating through the underlying vessel.

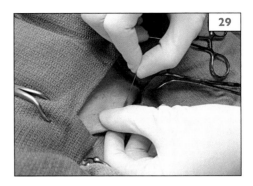

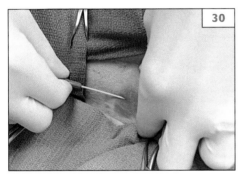

30 An assistant occludes venous outflow from the external jugular vein by placing pressure on the thoracic inlet. An over-the-needle catheter or hypodermic needle is inserted through the nick incision, into the underlying vessel.

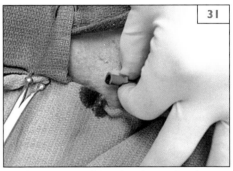

31 Once a flash of blood is observed in the catheter hub, the catheter is pushed into the vessel and the stylette removed. In most cases, blood will be observed flowing freely from the catheter hub, except in animals with extreme hypovolemia or hypotension.

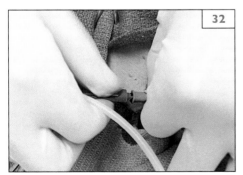

32 The hub of the J-wire introducer is inserted into the catheter hub, and the J-wire is pushed into the vessel.

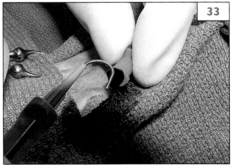

33 Once inside the vessel, the J wire will open up to its bent, characteristic 'J' shape, which prevents the tip of the wire from penetrating through a vessel or atrium wall.

The J-wire is then pushed into the vessel for almost its entire length, taking care to not let go of the wire (**34**). Once the J-wire is seated in the vessel, the catheter or needle is removed from over the wire, leaving only the wire seated in the vessel (**35**). The vascular dilator is pushed over the wire, through the skin and into the vessel with a brisk twisting motion (**36**). The vascular dilator does not need to be seated in the vessel up to its hub, but rather is used to make a larger hole in the vessel through which the catheter will be placed. Once a 'pop' is felt as the vascular dilator enters the vessel, the vascular dilator can be removed and the catheter inserted. It should be noted that once the vascular dilator is removed, the vessel will bleed, sometimes profusely. This is normal, as there is now a large hole in the vessel! The catheter and all catheter ports are flushed with heparinized saline, making sure that the catheter and attached lines are clear of any air bubbles before infusion. Infusion of a large air bubble can potentially be life-threatening and airlock the right ventricle, making forward blood flow, and hence life, impossible.

The vascular dilator is removed from the vessel and over the wire, and the catheter is

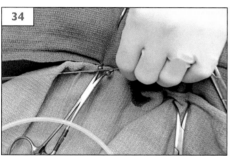

34 The over-the-needle catheter is pulled out of the vessel and off the J-wire. This leaves the J-wire seated in the vessel. The J-wire is pushed into the vessel for almost its entire length, but the end of the wire must be grasped once it becomes visible.

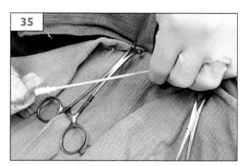

35 The vascular dilator is inserted over the wire, by holding the vascular dilator close to the skin, and pushing it into the vessel with a twisting motion.

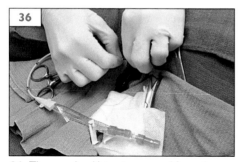

36 The vascular dilator is removed from the vessel and off the J-wire, and a flushed catheter is inserted over the wire, into the vessel.

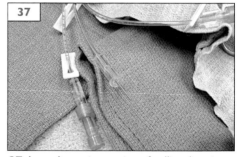

37 In an alternating motion of pulling the wire out slightly and pushing the catheter, the J-wire will eventually be visible from one of the proximal catheter ports. At this point, the wire should be grasped and the catheter pushed into the vessel.

then threaded over the J-wire. In many instances the catheter will be placed over the wire by alternating pushing of the catheter and pulling of the J-wire. The J-wire will eventually be observed in one of the proximal ports of the catheter (**37**). Once the J-wire can be grabbed from the proximal catheter port, the catheter is inserted to its length into the vessel. In some cases, the proper catheter placement can be predetermined by the catheter length and patient size. In other cases, the catheter should be inserted to an appropriate length, and then coiled on the outside of the patient to avoid pushing it in too far, for example into the heart (in the case of a jugular catheter). Most over-the-wire catheters have small holes in the proximal catheter port through which suture can be passed, then secured to the adjacent skin (**38**). The catheter is sutured in place, and bandaged to prevent contamination of the catheter entry site (**39**).

Peel-away catheters

Some manufacturers produce catheters that are introduced into a vessel with an over-the-needle catheter. Once the long catheter is seated within the vessel, the outer sheath of the catheter that was used to acquire vascular access is peeled away and the needle removed from the vessel, leaving only the long catheter in place. While this technique is technically easy, the choice of manufacturer often depends on operator preference and cost.

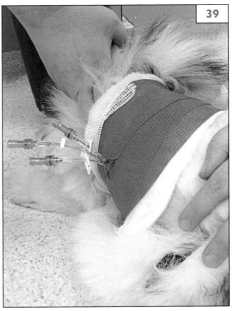

39 Lengths of cotton gauze and bandaging material are placed over the catheter entry site to prevent contamination.

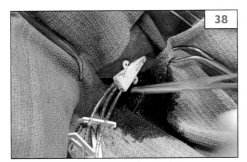

38 The catheter is sutured into place.

INTRAOSSEOUS CATHETERIZATION

Intraosseous catheters should be considered when vascular access is impossible due to small body size, anatomy (exotic patients), obesity, severe dehydration, hypotension, hypovolemia, or hypothermia.[3,4] As a general rule, any substance, including blood, parenteral nutrition products, and hyperosmolar solutions, that can be infused through an intravenous catheter can be infused through an intraosseous catheter, at rates equal to those through the intravenous catheter, including very fast or 'shock' rates of fluids.[3,4] Contraindications to placing an intraosseous catheter include abrasion or infection at the site of insertion, or bone fracture at the site of insertion. Several sites can be considered for intraosseous catheter placement, including the wing of the ileum, the femur, tibia, and proximal humerus (**40, 41** Depending on the size of the patient, spinal needles, hypodermic needles, or bone marrow needles can be placed as an intraosseous catheter (**42**). In an animal that is conscious, infusion of a local anesthetic to the level of the periosteum, in conjunction with systemic analgesic drugs, should be administered prior to catheter placement, to avoid discomfort.

To place an intraosseous catheter, the proposed catheter site is first clipped and aseptically scrubbed. The clinician should then palpate for the greater trochanter of the femur, and, holding the catheter in their dominant hand, gently push the catheter stylette through the skin and into the underlying intertrochanteric fossa with a simultaneous pushing and twisting motion (**43**). Once the needle is through the first cortex of the bone, the operator should feel less resistance as the needle passes into the marrow cavity. The catheter can be flushed with heparinized or nonheparinized saline. The saline solution should flow easily through the catheter. If the flush solution does not flow easily, two things must be considered: either the catheter is not in its proper place, or the catheter is clogged with bony debris. Pieces of bony debris will often occlude the catheter. Spinal needles or bone marrow biopsy needles that have an inner core can prevent occlusion of the catheter with

bone. In cases where a hypodermic needle has been placed, as in catheterization of a very small neonate or pocket pet, for example, the clogged needle should be removed and an identical needle placed in its place. A t-port is then secured to the hub of the needle or catheter (**44**). The t-port is then secured to the skin by a length of butterfly tape, or simply with a length of suture tied to the t-port, then used as if it were an intravenous catheter. Correct placement should be confirmed radiographically prior to use (**45**). Because intraosseous catheters can be uncomfortable, the catheter should be changed to an intravenous catheter whenever possible. Potential complications of intraosseous catheter placement include infection, nerve damage, fracture of the associated bone, embolism, and extravasation of the infused fluid.[3]

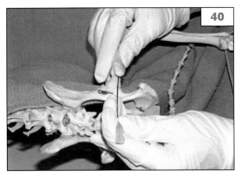

40 Demonstration on a skeleton of adducting the stifle and abducting the proximal femur, to open up the area around the intertrochanteric fossa of the femur, the point of intraosseous catheter placement.

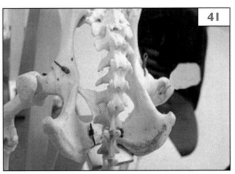

41 Placement of a spinal needle in the femur of a dog skeleton.

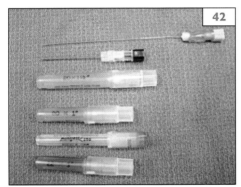

42 Types of needles that can be used for intraosseous catheterization include spinal needles with a stylette, or hypodermic needles for smaller patients and nonossified bones.

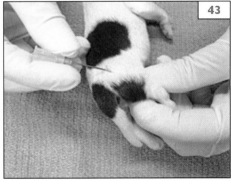

43 The distal femur is adducted toward the ventral midline and the hypodermic needle pushed through the skin, into the groove or intertrochanteric fossa of the femur, in a pushing/twisting motion.

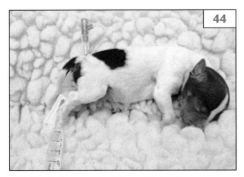

44 Final placement of the catheter in a puppy.

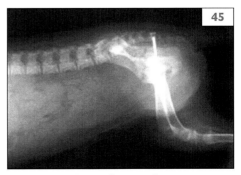

45 Radiographic verification of intraosseous catheter placement.

ARTERIAL CATHETERIZATION

Arterial catheterization should be considered whenever continuous blood pressure monitoring or frequent arterial blood sample collection is necessary.[6] Contraindications to catheterization of an artery include coagulopathies, infection over the proposed site of catheter placement, and in some cases, thromboembolic disease. Common sites for arterial catheterization include the dorsal pedal, auricular, femoral, and coccygeal arteries. The dorsal pedal artery is less prone to catheter dislodgement with patient movement, embolism and avascular necrosis of the extremity distal to the arterial catheter site, and contamination, and so is the preferred location whenever possible.[6]

The supplies required for placement of an arterial catheter are similar to those required for a peripheral intravenous catheter, and include a clean clipper with blades, antimicrobial scrub and antimicrobial solution, gauze 4 × 4 inch (100 × 100 mm) squares, 0.5 inch (12 mm) and 1 inch (24 mm) surgical adhesive tape, bandage material, heparinized saline flush, 3 mL syringe, and a flushed t-port.

The patient is first restrained in position. The auricular artery, pedal artery, and coccygeal artery are typically catheterized when a patient is under anesthesia, and are used short-term during the peri-anesthetic period. The dorsal pedal artery can be catheterized for longer use. For catheterization of the dorsal pedal artery, the animal is placed in lateral recumbency, with the limb that is going to be catheterized nearer to the table. The limb is extended and an assistant restrains the limb at the level of the hock or stifle, to prevent patient movement. The area over the dorsal pedal artery is clipped and aseptically scrubbed. The artery is palpated as it runs between the metatarsal bones (**46**). The stylette of an over-the-needle catheter is inserted through the skin at an approximately 15–30° angle (**47**), and is pushed into the artery until a flash of blood is seen in the catheter hub. If a flash is not observed, the stylette should be advanced in millimeter increments to catheterize the artery. Once a flash of blood is observed (**48**) the stylette and catheter are advanced an additional 1–2 mm, and the catheter is pushed into the artery. Once the catheter is seated properly in the artery, pulsatile blood can be observed in the catheter

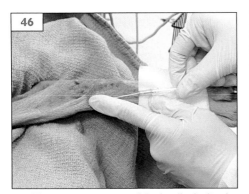

46 The anterior portion of the hindlimb, distal to the tarsus, over the metatarsal bones, is palpated for a pulse from the dorsal pedal artery.

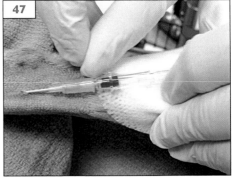

47 After insertion of the catheter into the artery, a flash of blood will be observed in the catheter hub. The catheter is pushed off the stylette, into the artery.

hub (**49**). Several gauze squares should then be secured under the catheter hub to prevent iatrogenic contamination of the site with blood, and to keep the area dry to facilitate tape adhering to the skin. A length of 0.5 inch (12 mm) white adhesive surgical tape is secured around the hub of the catheter, and around the distal limb, followed by a length of 1 inch (24 mm) tape under the catheter hub to secure the catheter in place. A third length of tape can be placed over the catheter hub and around the distal limb. The catheter is then flushed with heparinized saline (**50**). Technically, at this point, the catheter is ready for use. Many clinicians will also secure bandage material around the catheter, and label the catheter and line carefully to prevent the catheter from being used for anything other than blood pressure monitoring or arterial blood sample removal (**51**).[6,7]

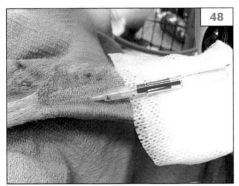

48 Example of a catheter placed in the dorsal pedal artery. After placement, a piece of gauze is placed under the catheter hub, to prevent soiling the underlying skin and fur, which could prevent the tape from adhering securely to the skin.

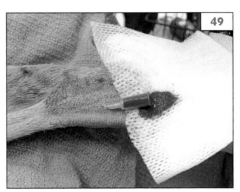

49 Pulsatile blood flows freely when the catheter is placed in the artery.

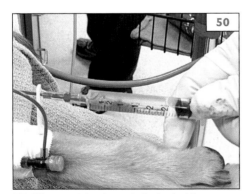

50 The arterial catheter is flushed with heparinized saline.

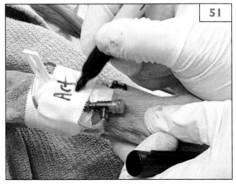

51 An arterial catheter should always be labeled 'Not for IV infusion'.

VASCULAR CUTDOWN

Vascular access may be very difficult in animals that are severely dehydrated, hypovolemic, hypotensive, hypothermic, obese, or have peripheral edema.[2,7] In such instances, it may also be difficult to place an intraosseous catheter, particularly in large adult or obese animals. For this reason, veterinary personnel should be adept at performing vascular cutdowns when necessary in the emergent situation.

Supplies necessary to perform an emergent vascular cutdown should be secured in a sterile surgical pack and within hand's reach on the rare instance that an emergency requires it. It is a good idea to keep a surgical pack in the same area as the crash cart. Each surgical pack should contain a scalpel handle, scalpel blade, curved and straight hemostats and mosquito hemostat forceps, thumb forceps, absorbable suture (3-0), Mayo and Metzenbaum scissors, gauze 4 × 4 inch (100 × 100 mm) squares, and field towels.

Any vessel that can have a peripheral catheter placed within it by percutaneous means is a candidate for having a catheter placed via vascular cutdown. The jugular, cephalic, and lateral saphenous veins are easy to locate and catheterize because of their size and location.[5]

To perform an emergent vascular cutdown, the proposed catheter placement site is clipped and aseptically scrubbed. The area should be draped with sterile field towels, to prevent contamination of the catheter site. A small amount of local anesthetic is injected under the skin over the proposed site of catheter insertion, taking care to avoid injecting the local anesthetic directly into the vessel (**52**). Next, the skin over the vessel is picked up with a thumb forceps, and a skin incision made over the vessel, taking care to avoid lacerating the underlying vessel and tissues (**53**). The incision must be large enough to be able to visualize structures and identify the vessel. The underlying tissue is bluntly dissected to the level of the vessel (**54**). It is extremely important that all of the connective tissue fascia that surrounds the vessel is removed. Using a mosquito hemostat, two individual stay sutures are placed under the vessel, and secured with a

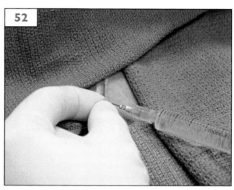

52 The skin is tented and the area over the vessel infiltrated with local anesthetic, such as 0.5–1 mg/kg lidocaine.

hemostat forceps (**55**). An assistant should then lift the vessel up, so that it is parallel with the skin incision (**56**) and the catheter is inserted into the vessel, taking care to avoid pushing the catheter through the vessel. Once the catheter is seated in the vessel, the absorbable stay sutures can be used to secure the catheter gently in the vessel (**57**). The suture should not be too tight, as at some point the catheter will have to be removed from the vessel. The skin is then sutured over the catheter as for any other skin incision (**58**) and the catheter secured in position with tape in the same manner as if the catheter was placed percutaneously. Once a catheter can be placed percutaneously, the catheter placed via vascular cutdown should be removed, as the risk of contamination and infection is greater than when a catheter is placed in a nonemergent situation.

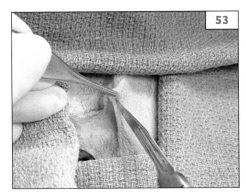

53 The skin is incised over the vessel with a scalpel blade, taking care to avoid lacerating the underlying vessel.

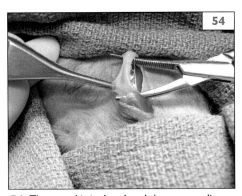

54 The vessel is isolated, and the surrounding fascia/connective tissue bluntly dissected to expose the vessel.

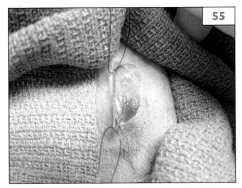

55 Two absorbable stay sutures are placed under the vessel. This allows lifting of the vessel to the level of the skin to facilitate catheter placement.

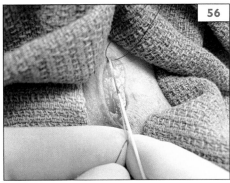

56 The catheter is inserted into the vessel, taking care to avoid penetrating through the back wall of the vessel.

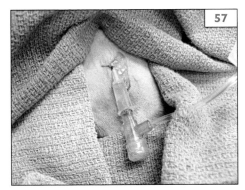

57 Once the catheter is seated in the vessel the absorbable suture can be loosely secured around the catheter.

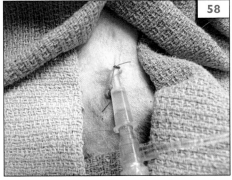

58 The skin is sutured over the catheter, and the catheter hub taped as previously described for a percutaneously placed catheter.

THE THREE-SYRINGE BLOOD SAMPLING TECHNIQUE

The 'three-syringe' technique is one used to obtain unadulterated blood samples from a peripheral or central venous catheter, and then to administer the heparinized blood back to the patient. Nonsterile gloves should be worn, to prevent catheter contamination. Three syringes are prepared, including a 3 mL or 6 mL syringe into which 0.5 mL of heparinized saline has been drawn. The male adapter or intravenous tubing is disconnected, and the male end of the heparinized syringe is inserted into the female end of the catheter hub, and 3 mL or 6 mL of blood are slowly withdrawn (the amount varies depending on whether the catheter is peripheral or central). The heparinized blood sample should be capped with a hypodermic needle, to prevent contamination. An unadulterated blood sample is then similarly collected into a sterile syringe, and the sample decanted into the appropriate collection tube. The heparinized blood sample is then administered back into the venous, not the arterial catheter, and the catheter flushed with 3 mL or 6 mL of heparinized saline from a third syringe.

MAINTENANCE OF THE INTRAVENOUS CATHETER

Intravenous catheter maintenance is as important as catheter placement technique to prevent contamination of the catheter site and avoid an iatrogenic nosocomial infection. One of the most important aspects in preventing catheter contamination is first to identify conditions which could potentially cause catheter contamination, such as vomiting, diarrhea, or urinary incontinence. The catheter should be placed in a location where it will be less likely to become contaminated by the patient's body fluids. The catheter should be monitored at least twice to three times daily for evidence of surrounding redness, swelling, or pain upon injection that could indicate phlebitis, infection, or thrombosis.[2]

Whenever a catheter and fluid lines are handled, hospital personnel should wash their hands carefully with antiseptic scrub or lotion, and then wear gloves to prevent catheter contamination. Bandages should be changed as soon as strikethrough or soiling is observed.[2] As a general rule, as long as the catheter is patent and has not developed any of the complications listed above and the patient remains afebrile, the catheter can be used. Frequent catheter changes do not reduce the incidence of bacterial infection, but have been shown to significantly increase the patient's hospital bill.

COMPLICATIONS ASSOCIATED WITH INTRAVENOUS CATHETERIZATION

Contamination of the catheter site from the patient's body fluids and excrement, or from invasion of nosocomial organisms in the hospital environment, is one of the most common causes of catheter-induced complications. In the hospital environment, transfer of nosocomial organisms from instruments and the hands of personnel can be a significant source of infection (**59**). Elizabethan collars prevent chewing of the catheter or intravenous fluid line (**60**). Additionally, breaks in sterility of the catheter or fluid line can increase the likelihood of catheter-related infection.

Large-bore central venous catheters are relatively contraindicated in any animal with a hyper- or hypocoagulable state. For example, the placement of a large-bore central catheter in an animal with disseminated intravascular coagulation (DIC) or the vitamin K antagonist rodenticide intoxication can be associated with unnecessary iatrogenic hemorrhage from the catheter site. Conditions associated with hypercoagulability, such as immune-mediated hemolytic anemia, hyperadrenocorticism, DIC, or protein-losing enteropathies or nephropathies, can be associated with an increased risk of thromboembolism. Thrombosis of the cranial vena cava has been reported secondary to jugular vein catheterization.[8]

Aseptic techniques should be used at all times during placement and maintenance of an intravenous catheter to reduce the risk of bacterial contamination of the catheter site. One of the most common sources of catheter-induced infection, besides the animals themselves, is from the equipment and hands of the hospital personnel. Hand-washing is by far one of the most important tasks that a veterinary technician and veterinarian can perform to prevent catheter-related infections. The incidence of catheter-related infection in one veterinary critical care unit documented *Enterobacter* spp. contamination of intravenous catheters. In the same study, change of personnel resulted in a significant decrease in the incidence of catheter-related infection.[9] The lack of hygiene of certain personnel may have contributed significantly to positive bacterial cultures of intravenous catheters.

All personnel that place intravenous catheters should wear gloves during and after scrubbing the catheter site with an antimicrobial scrub solution. This is particularly important in immunocompromised animals, such as those with diabetes mellitus, cancer and chemotherapy, and parvoviral enteritis. In puppies with parvoviral enteritis, the incidence of bacterial contamination of catheters can be as high as 22%.[10] The majority of bacterial pathogens isolated were from either gastrointestinal or environmental sources, and were resistant to multiple antibiotics.[10] Because of the high incidence of bacterial resistance, a likely source of contamination was due to environmental pathogens, possibly due to transfer from the environment by the hands of the animal's caretakers. Another study documented that use of a 4% chlorhexidine scrub on a distal extremity, followed by a contact time of 1 minute, greatly reduced bacterial colonization of skin at intravenous catheter sites.[11] However, an intravenous catheter is frequently dragged through the fur on the patient's distal extremity prior to insertion into the vessel, causing contamination. To avoid this potential source of contamination of the catheter site, a gauze 4 × 4 inch (100 × 100 mm) square should be situated over the fur prior to placement of the intravenous catheter.

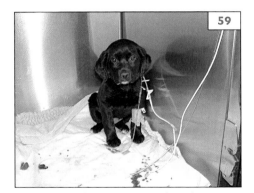

59 Example of contamination of a catheter site and intravenous fluid line with vomitus and diarrheic feces from a puppy with parvoviral enteritis.

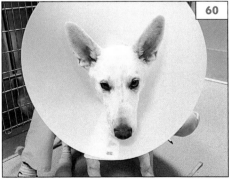

60 Elizabethan collars may be required to prevent a patient from chewing a catheter and associated bandage.

During emergency placement of intravenous or intraosseous catheters, nonsterile technique can contribute to catheter-related infection and complications. Even when strict adherence to aseptic protocols has been used, the catheter site should be checked at least once a day for evidence of pain upon injection, erythema, 'ropiness' or thickening of the vessel, heat, or any discharge from the catheter site. If any of these abnormalities are noted, or if a fever develops in a previously afebrile patient, the catheter should be removed and the catheter tip cultured for aerobic bacteria (**61**).

It was once considered to be a gold standard to remove and replace an intravenous catheter routinely every 3 days, even if the catheter was still patent and not causing any problem. More recent evidence has demonstrated that there is no increased risk of catheter-related complications, including bacterial contamination, if an intravenous catheter remains in place for longer than 72 hours.[12] Animals that had catheters in place for longer than 72 hours did not have a significantly different risk of bacterial contamination, and in fact, the overall risk of bacterial contamination was low. Bacteria that were cultured from the catheters included *Enterobacter aerogenes*, *Staphylococcus aureus*, *Pseudomonas aeruginosa*, *Pasteurella multocida*, and *Bacillus* spp. Interestingly, the authors found that gauze sponges were a source of *Bacillus* spp. contamination. The incidence of catheter-related infection significantly decreased once the source of contamination was found and removed. Therefore, careful maintenance of supplies used in the placement and maintenance of intravenous catheters is also important, and may be an inadvertently overlooked source of infection, if complications arise.

Another study documented that length of time since catheter placement was not correlated with the incidence of bacterial infection or other catheter-related complications.[9] In one observational study of human patients with more than 600 catheters, there was no increased risk of infection, thrombophlebitis, or mechanical complications associated with prolonged catheterization.[13] For these reasons, therefore, as long as a catheter is necessary and works without problems, newer recommendations suggest that it is not necessary to replace the catheter so frequently, unless problems arise. However, if fever, pain upon injection, or thrombophlebitis occur, the catheter must be removed and the catheter tip cultured. As a general rule, once the catheter is no longer needed it should be removed as soon as possible, as it can always be a potential source of infection and thrombophlebitis.

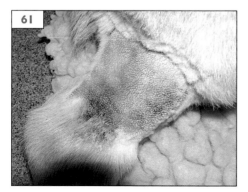

61 An example of a catheter site that has become bruised. The underlying vessel had developed thrombosis and felt thickened. Pain was elicited upon infusion into the catheter, so it was removed.

Components of crystalloid fluids and potential complications of fluid therapy

- **Introduction**

- **Constituents of crystalloid fluids**

- **Complications of intravenous fluid therapy**

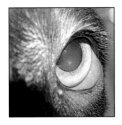
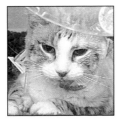
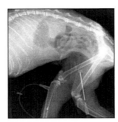
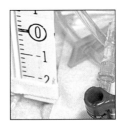

INTRODUCTION

When choosing a fluid for the treatment of a specific disease, the caregiver must carefully consider the animal's primary and secondary diseases, the metabolic and acid–base status, and the presence of underlying conditions such as cardiac or renal insufficiency or vasculitis that can influence the animal's ability to respond appropriately, rather than adversely, to therapy. Ideally, the choice of which crystalloid fluid to administer for a particular disease is analogous to choosing an antibiotic for various types of bacterial infections.

A crystalloid fluid is basically a solution of water with various forms of electrolyte or salt or sugar crystals (**62**).[1] Crystalloid fluids are categorized according to their osmolality relative to plasma. Electrolytes can move across a semipermeable membrane or barrier by the process of osmosis (**63**).[1,2] In many cases, an electrolyte will move down a concentration gradient from an area of higher concentration to an area of lower concentration. Therefore, the concentration of osmotically active particles in a crystalloid fluid will influence the amount of fluid that is retained within the intravascular compartment after intravenous aministration.

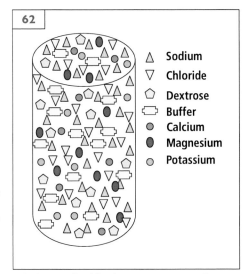

62 A crystalloid fluid contains water and various concentrations of sodium, chloride and/or dextrose particles. Other components which may or may not be present in different concentrations include potassium, magnesium, calcium, and a buffer. Depending on the type of fluid, the buffer is either lactate, acetate, or gluconate.

63 Diagram of osmosis. The large orange particles are present in a higher concentration on the left side of the semipermeable membrane. Water is in a relatively higher concentration on the right side of the semipermeable membrane. The pores in the semipermeable membrane are freely permeable to water, but not to larger particles. Water is allowed to flow down its concentration gradient (higher concentration on the right side and lower concentration on the left side) over to the left side of the membrane until equal amounts of water are on either side of the membrane. The larger particles are not allowed to cross from one side to the other.

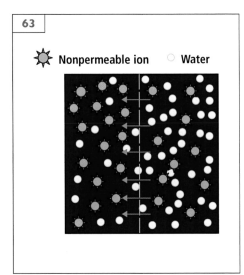

An isotonic crystalloid fluid has an osmolality equal to that of plasma and the extracellular compartment. Fluids with tonicity lower than that of the extracellular space are called hypotonic, and can cause fluid influx into red blood cells and hence hemolysis.[1,2] Fluids with tonicity greater than that of the extracellular fluid compartment are called hypertonic, and can be used to expand intravascular fluid volume in a hypovolemic animal. Approximately 80% of isotonic crystalloid fluids will leave the intravascular compartment and move to the interstitial compartment within 1 hour of administration, unless measures such as concurrent intravenous administration of a colloid are also performed.[3]

Intravenous fluids can be used for a variety of reasons, including re-expansion of intravascular fluid volume, rehydration of the interstitial and intracellular compartments, maintenance and correction of acid–base and electrolyte disorders, and to establish and maintain vascular access (*Table 8*).[4]

Table 8
Relative indications and contraindications for use of isotonic, hypotonic, and hypertonic crystalloid fluids

Fluid	Indications	Relative contraindications
Normosol-R	Replacement, metabolic acidosis, anorexia, vomiting, hypovolemic shock, diarrhea, renal failure	Hyperkalemia, metabolic alkalosis
Plasmalyte-A	Replacement, metabolic acidosis, anorexia, vomiting, hypovolemic shock, diarrhea, renal failure	Hyperkalemia, metabolic alkalosis
0.9% NaCl	Replacement, hypovolemic shock, anorexia, vomiting, diarrhea, metabolic alkalosis, hyperkalemia, hypercalcemia, hyponatremia, renal failure	Cardiac disease, liver disease, metabolic acidosis
Lactated Ringer's	Replacement, hypovolemic shock, vomiting, anorexia, diarrhea, hypocalcemia, metabolic acidosis, renal failure	Hypercalcemia, hyperkalemia, blood product administration, liver failure
5% Dextrose in water	Drug carrier, correction of hypernatremia and free water deficit, congestive heart failure	Does not provide sufficient calories to be used as a form of parenteral nutrition
0.45% NaCl + 2.5% dextrose	Maintenance, replacement of insensible losses, correction of free water deficit	Not to be used as a replacement fluid; hyponatremia; not to be used for shock resuscitation
Normosol-M	Replacement of insensible losses	Hyponatremia; not to be used as a replacement fluid; not to be used for shock resuscitation

(*Continued*)

Table 8
Relative indications and contraindication for use of isotonic, hypotonic, and hypertonic crystalloid fluids (*Continued*)

Fluid	Indications	Relative contraindications
Plasmalyte-M	Replacement of insensible losses	Hyponatremia; not to be used as a replacement fluid; not to be used for shock resuscitation
3% NaCl	Intravascular volume expansion, hypovolemic shock	Interstitial dehydration, hypernatremia
7% NaCl	Intravascular volume expansion, hypovolemic shock	Interstitial dehydration, hypernatremia

Table 9
Constituents of crystalloid solutions

Fluid	Osmolality	Buffer	Sodium	Chloride	Potassium
Normosol-R	296	Acetate 27 Gluconate 23	140	98	5
Plasmalyte-A	294	Acetate 27 Gluconate 23	140	98	5
0.9% Saline	308	0	154	154	0
Lactated Ringer's	272	Lactate 28	130	109	4
5% Dextrose in water	252	0	0	0	0
0.45% NaCl + 2.5% dextrose	280	0	77	77	0
Normosol-M + 2.5% dextrose	363	Acetate 16	40	40	13
Plasmalyte-M + 5% dextrose	377	Acetate 12 Lactate 12	40	40	16
3% NaCl	1026	0	513	513	0
7% NaCl	2400	0	1283	1283	0

The specific type of intravenous fluid that is chosen for a particular disease should be based on its individual components (*Table 9*). In addition to being categorized based on the tonicity relative to the extracellular compartment, intravenous fluids are also categorized for their role in either replacing or maintaining serum acid–base and electrolyte status, or in the retention of fluid within the vascular space.

Intravenous fluids are also classified according to their role in the replacement of intravascular or interstitial fluid or electrolyte deficits, or to maintain electrolyte balance. A balanced crystalloid fluid is one that contains components very similar to those of the extracellular space.[5] Unbalanced crystalloid solutions are lacking in one or more components found in the extracellular space.[5] Replacement crystalloid solutions contain components similar to those of the extracellular space.[5] In general, isotonic crystalloid fluids for replacement of fluid and electrolyte deficits have sodium concentrations similar to those of plasma and the extracellular fluid compartment[1,2,4] Several solutions are used for replacement of fluid volume, electrolyte abnormalities, and correction of acid–base abnormalities, including Normosol-R, Plasmalyte-A, normal (0.9%) saline and lactated Ringer's. This list is not exhaustive, and the reader should use the information and concepts discussed here to assess the crystalloid fluids available locally.

Maintenance crystalloid solutions contain lower concentrations of sodium and other compounds than the extracellular space,[1,2,5] and are used primarily to replace sensible and insensible fluid losses.[3] An example of a maintenance isotonic crystalloid fluid is 0.45% sodium with 2.5% dextrose (also known as 'half-strength saline with dextrose'). Other important components of isotonic crystalloid fluids to consider include buffers, calcium, magnesium, potassium, and chloride (*Table 9*).

Calcium	Magnesium	Glucose
0	3	0
0	3	0
0	0	0
3	0	0
0	0	50 g/L
0	0	25 g/L
0	3	50 g/L
5	3	100 g/L
0	0	0
0	0	0

CONSTITUENTS OF CRYSTALLOID FLUIDS

Buffers

A buffer is a compound that is converted or metabolized in the body to bicarbonate. Bicarbonate is a major buffer within the body that helps control the pH of the blood. Lactate is a buffer that is converted to bicarbonate by a normally functioning liver. In cases of hepatic dysfunction, however, the liver's ability to convert lactate to bicarbonate may be diminished. In such cases, use of a crystalloid that contains acetate or gluconate, which are both converted to bicarbonate in muscle, is preferred. In some cases, such as anesthetic-induced hypotension, some practitioners avoid acetate-containing solutions owing to their belief that acetate will potentiate hypotension.

Lactated Ringer's solutions contain lactate as the primary buffer. Other crystalloid fluids such as Plasmalyte- (-A, 148, -M, and 56) contain acetate as the primary buffer. Medical conditions which cause metabolic acidosis should ideally be treated with a crystalloid fluid that contains some buffer that will be metabolized ultimately to bicarbonate.

Infusion of the intravenous fluid will first cause volume expansion and hopefully improve perfusion, such that lactate and other by-products of anaerobic metabolism are diluted. The buffers contained within the crystalloid fluid will be converted into bicarbonate and increase serum pH. With a condition such as diabetic acidosis, however, normal (0.9%) saline has been recommended as the fluid of choice to replace intravascular circulating volume. As insulin and dextrose are administered, ketoacids present will also be converted to bicarbonate, raising the serum pH. As a general rule, severe metabolic acidosis with a venous pH <7.1 warrants therapeutic intervention with bicarbonate supplementation in addition to that being provided by the buffered isotonic crystalloid fluid solution. The patient's bicarbonate deficit can be calculated and then administered as sodium bicarbonate, using the following equation:

Bicarbonate deficit (mEq/L)
  = Base deficit × 0.4 × body weight (kg)

Because the infusion of the buffered isotonic crystalloid will promote volume expansion and dilute the acidosis present in the patient, a conservative method of replenishing bicarbonate stores is to calculate the bicarbonate deficit, then administer one-third of the calculated value as a slow bolus, then the rest over a 24 hour period. Overzealous administration of bicarbonate can potentially cause a paradoxical cerebrospinal acidosis and a metabolic alkalosis, both of which are difficult to treat. For this reason, some practitioners recommend not supplementing with sodium bicarbonate unless the pH remains <7.2 after appropriate intravenous fluid resuscitation. Normal (0.9%) saline contains no buffers, and is known as an acidifying crystalloid fluid because it will promote excretion of bicarbonate by the renal tubules.[4] In cases of metabolic alkalosis, such as that observed with an upper gastrointestinal obstruction, an acidifying solution such as 0.9% saline without additional buffers is preferred, in order to avoid the administration of additional sources of bicarbonate, and also to replenish chloride ions lost in vomitus.

Sodium concentration

Sodium is the major extracellular cation in the body. Normal sodium concentrations are 140–150 mEq/L for dogs and 150–160 mEq/L for cats.[4] The sodium content of most isotonic crystalloid fluids ranges from 130 mEq/L to 154 mEq/L.

Rapid changes in serum sodium concentration can be detrimental, depending on how quickly an animal's sodium balance and serum sodium concentration become deranged. Hypernatremia is largely characterized by a free water deficit, i.e. a deficit of fluid in excess of electrolytes. Diarrhea, heat-induced illness, hyperthermia, and lack of access to water can cause varying degrees of hypernatremia. In contrast, syndromes such as hypoadrenocorticism, pseudohypoadreno-corticism, and abdominal or pleural effusions can cause decreases in serum sodium concentration, or hyponatremia. Ideally, serum sodium concentration should not be lowered or raised by more than 15 mEq in a 24 hour period. Overzealous administration of sodium-containing fluids such as normal (0.9%) saline to treat severe hyponatremia can result in cerebral edema and central pontine myelinolysis.[6]

Conditions that promote hyperaldosteronemia and sodium retention, such as congestive heart failure and hepatic failure, may benefit from infusion of fluids with lower concentrations of sodium, such as 0.45% sodium chloride (NaCl), or 5% dextrose in water.

Fluids used to replace intravascular and interstitial volume deficit should contain 130–154 mEq/L of sodium. Normal (0.9%) saline is the crystalloid fluid with the highest sodium concentration (154 mEq/L), and lactated Ringers contains the lowest concentration of sodium (130 mEq/L) relative to plasma.

Maintenance fluids can be used to replace daily ongoing sodium losses. Fluids such as Plasmalyte-M and Plasmalyte 56 contain approximately 40 mEq/L sodium. If such fluids were used as replacement solutions, the patient's serum sodium could decrease and lead to a state of hyponatremia.

Hypertonic saline contains supraphysiologic concentrations of sodium, and is largely used to expand intravascular fluid volume by extracting fluid from the interstitial space. As the name implies, hypertonic saline has a tonicity (1712 mOsm/L in 5%, 2567 mOsm/L in 7.5%) much higher than that of serum/plasma. Infusion of hypertonic saline makes plasma hypertonic to the surrounding interstitium, so fluid moves from the interstitium into the intravascular space to reduce the relative increase in serum osmolality (**64**).

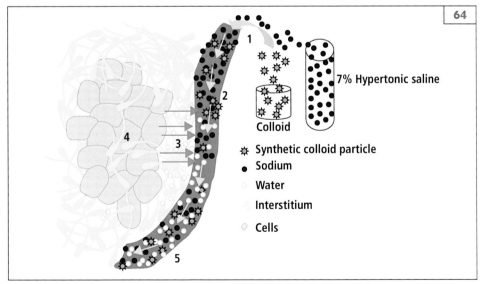

64 An intravenous infusion of hypertonic saline (Step 1) loads the vasculature with a large number of osmotically active particles such that the intravascular space becomes hyperosmolar in relation to the interstitium and the cells (Step 2). By the process of osmosis, fluid leaves the interstitial (Step 3), then the intracellular compartments (Step 4) in an attempt to normalize serum osmolality. The net movement of interstitial and intracellular water into the vascular space transiently increases intravascular fluid volume. Once serum osmolality is diluted and becomes equilibrated towards normal (Step 5), the fluid within the vascular space will move back into the interstitial and intracellular compartments unless the hypertonic saline is infused along with a colloid. The colloid protects and maintains the fluid load within the intravascular compartment to maintain circulating blood volume. Because the interstitium and intracellular space are now effectively dehydrated, boluses of hypertonic saline and colloid should be followed by administration of an isotonic crystalloid fluid so that the balance of fluids between all compartments is normalized.

This can create a relative increase in the tonicity of the interstitial space, and pull fluid from the intracellular compartment. In order to replenish the interstitial deficit caused by the administration of hypertonic saline, an isotonic crystalloid fluid also should be administered. Re-equilibration of the intravascular crystalloid fluid administered later allows normalization of interstitial and intracellular fluid deficits.[1] Because hypertonic saline induces intravascular volume expansion by pulling fluid from the interstitial and intracellular fluid compartments, its infusion is contraindicated in animals with interstitial dehydration or hypernatremia.[7] The intravascular volume expansion effects of hypertonic saline are relatively short-lived (approximately 20 minutes), so the fluid should be infused along with a synthetic colloid to achieve more sustained effects. Ideally, hypertonic saline in combination with a colloid (5–10 mL/kg in dogs, 2 mL/kg in cats) should be infused slowly over 15 minutes as a single dose, to avoid hypotension.[4]

Chloride

Chloride is a major extracellular anion. Chloride can be lost in vomitus caused by an upper gastrointestinal obstruction, or can be lost in diarrheic feces. Metabolic derangements characteristic of an upper gastrointestinal obstruction include hypochloremic metabolic alkalosis. Normal (0.9%) saline contains supraphysiologic concentrations of chloride (154 mEq/L), and is used as a chloride replacement fluid in cases of hypochloremia. Other isotonic crystalloid fluids contain varying concentrations of chloride (55–103 mEq/L). While chloride is important, consideration of sodium and other electrolyte concentrations is more important when selecting a replacement fluid for a specific disease state.

Potassium

Potassium is the major intracellular anion. Serum potassium can become elevated due to severe dehydration, hypoadrenocorticism, metabolic acidosis, diabetic ketoacidosis, and renal failure. Renal insufficiency can also result in varying degrees of hypokalemia. Most replacement and maintenance crystalloid fluids contain some form of supplemental potassium. In animals with hyperkalemia, it is best to avoid the administration of a potassium-containing fluid whenever possible. Administration of intravenous fluids alone, however, will dilute serum potassium as intravascular fluid volume is replenished, even if the fluid contains small amounts of potassium. In animals with hypokalemia, potassium supplementation is commensurate with the degree of hypokalemia (*Table 10*).[8] It is advisable not to administer more than 0.5 mEq/kg/hr potassium intravenously (*Table 11*).

Magnesium is required for regulation and normal functioning of the sodium–potassium–ATPase pump. In animals with refractory hypokalemia, as seen in some animals with diabetic ketoacidosis, for example, magnesium should be supplemented (0.75 mEq/kg/day) in addition to potassium.

Table 10
Recommended doses for potassium supplementation in hypokalemia

Serum potassium (mEq/L)	Potassium (mEq) to be added to 1L of fluids
≤2.0	80
2.1–2.5	60
2.6–3.0	40
3.1–3.5	30
3.6–5.0	20
>6.0*	0

*Should strongly consider supplementing with a crystalloid fluid that does not contain potassium and will promote potassium excretion. An ideal choice would be 0.9% NaCl.

Table 11
Potassium supplementation (mEq/L) and maximum rate of fluid administration (mL/kg/hr) to avoid exceeding the recommended 0.5 mEq/kg/hr potassium infusion IV

Potassium supplementation (mEq/L)	Maximum rate of fluid administration (mL/kg/hr)
80	6.25
70	7.1
60	8.3
40	12.5
30	16.7
20	25

Calcium

Calcium is an important ion that is necessary for normal muscle conduction and coagulation. Calcium is present in small amounts in lactated Ringer's (3 mEq/L) solution. In cases of puerperal tetany (eclampsia), for example, lactated Ringer's may be the preferred fluid to administer in addition to treatment with 10% calcium gluconate or calcium chloride. Some conditions, such as an intentional or unintentional removal of the parathyroid gland(s) during a parathyroidectomy or thyroidectomy, may predispose an animal to the development of hypocalcemia. In addition to standard medical protocols in such cases, the pre-emptive use of a calcium-containing fluid such as lactated Ringer's may be beneficial in helping to prevent hypocalcemia during the post-operative period. Hypercalcemia can be due to a variety of causes (*Table 12*).

Administration of a calcium-containing fluid is relatively contraindicated if other crystalloid fluids are available. Normal (0.9%) saline is the treatment of choice in cases of hypercalcemia, not only because the fluid does not contain calcium, but also because the saline promotes calciuresis.

Dextrose

Dextrose-containing fluids are largely hypotonic compared to plasma. D5W (5% dextrose in water) is analogous to a free water solution. Because water alone is severely hypotonic relative to plasma, infusion of free water will cause rapid and severe hemolysis of the red blood cells. The addition of 5% dextrose (50 mg dextrose/mL) brings the tonicity of the fluid into a safe acceptable range. Once infused, the dextrose is quickly metabolized and the remaining fluid redistributes within the intravascular, interstitial, and intracellular fluid compartments. Dextrose-containing fluids such as D5W and 0.45% NaCl with 2.5% dextrose are often used as maintenance fluids in the treatment of diabetic ketoacidosis, hepatic failure, cardiac disease, and for infusion of some drug products. In animals with hepatic and cardiac disease, relative hyperaldosteronism can cause sodium retention. Therefore, it is preferable to administer D5W or 0.45% NaCl + 2.5% dextrose, rather than add dextrose to an isotonic crystalloid that contains 130–154 mEq/L sodium. The dextrose in these fluids, in the concentrations listed, is quickly metabolized, but is largely insufficient to meet an animal's daily metabolic caloric requirements.

Table 12
Causes of hypercalcemia

GOSH DARN IT!

Granulomatous disease – blastomycosis and other fungal disease

Osteogenic – metastatic bone tumors

Spurious – laboratory error

Hyperparathyroidism

D Vitamin D toxicity/cholecalciferol rodenticide intoxication

Addison's disease/hypoadrenocorticism

Renal failure

Neoplasia – lymphoma, apocrine gland adenocarcinoma, multiple myeloma, leukemia, fibrosarcoma

Idiopathic (cats)

T Temperature and toxins – cholecalciferol rodenticides, calcium supplements

COMPLICATIONS OF INTRAVENOUS FLUID THERAPY

Intravascular volume overload

Total body water comprises an estimated 60% of the animal's body weight. Approximately 67% of the total body water is located intracellularly within cells, and the rest is located in the extracellular, intravascular and interstitial spaces. Of the 33% of water that is located extracellularly, 24% is located in the interstitial space, and 8–10% is located within the intravascular space. The flux, or movement, of fluid from one compartment to another is governed by a delicate balance between hydrostatic forces and oncotic forces within each compartment, as well as vascular endothelial pore size.

Hydrostatic force is the pressure that water exerts on either side of a blood vessel wall: that is, within the vessel, the intravascular hydrostatic pressure, and on the other side of the vessel wall, the interstitial hydrostatic pressure. Elevations in hydrostatic forces favor extravasation of fluid from one compartment to the other, if oncotic forces are suboptimal. Conversely, oncotic forces favor retention of fluid within a fluid compartment, helping to avoid interstitial edema if a healthy vasculature is present. Starling's Law of Diffusion[9] describes fluid flux, or the movement of fluid from one compartment to another, where:

$$\text{Fluid movement} = k[(P_c + \pi_i) - (\pi_c + P_i)]$$

where k = filtration coefficient, P_c = hydrostatic pressure in the capillary, P_i = hydrostatic pressure in the interstitium, π_c = capillary oncotic pressure, and π_i = oncotic pressure of the interstitial space.

The filtration coefficient is determined by the capillary fenestration or pore size. Oncotic pressure is the force that attracts fluid or water, and helps to retain fluid within a compartment. The oncotic pressure is determined by the size and number of particles in solution relative to the size and number of particles in the interstitial space. The capillary hydrostatic pressure and interstitial oncotic pressure influence movement of fluid into the interstitial space. Conversely, the capillary oncotic pressure and interstitial hydrostatic pressure favor fluid retention within the intravascular compartment. It is the balance between the forces favoring filtration and the forces driving fluid absorption that determines the net direction of fluid flux.

When intravascular hydrostatic pressure exceeds intravascular oncotic pressure, fluid can move into the interstitial compartment, resulting in interstitial edema. Crystalloid fluids have no oncotic pressure, and so can dilute serum colloid oncotic pressure (COP), albumin, and other serum proteins. Overzealous crystalloid fluid administration, particularly in the presence of hypoalbuminemia, increases the risk of interstitial edema.[1,2] This is particularly detrimental in the lungs: when pulmonary capillary pressures exceed 25 mmHg, pulmonary edema can occur, and the pulmonary lymphatic drainage system becomes overwhelmed.

Direct cardiac output monitoring with a pulmonary artery catheter and measurement of pulmonary capillary occlusion pressure is not advocated or widely available for use in all critically ill animals. Central venous pressure measurements, however, are simple and easy to perform with minimally invasive equipment, and can be used to measure indirect trends in intravascular fluid volume, provided that right heart function, vascular compliance, and intrathoracic pressures are normal.[10] Colloid osmometry is an additional monitoring tool that is useful to determine a patient's colloid oncotic pressure and response to colloid fluid therapy.[11] In the past, practitioners have attempted to extrapolate serum oncotic pressure from an animal's serum total protein; however, the results are variable, and do not correlate very well with direct measurements of COP.[12–14]

Intravascular oncotic pressure and fluid volume must be carefully titrated to meet the animal's fluid therapy needs. Consequences of edema include impaired cellular oxygen delivery and enzymatic functions, impaired cellular oxygen exchange, cellular swelling, and cell lysis.[8] Clinical signs associated with overhydration can include serous nasal discharge, chemosis, tachypnea, restlessness, cough, pulmonary crackles, and shivering. Tachypnea and cough often occur before clinical signs of serous nasal discharge, chemosis (**65**), peripheral edema (**66**), or fulminant pulmonary edema (**67**). Therefore, frequent assessment of the animal's respiratory status is an important component of patient monitoring.

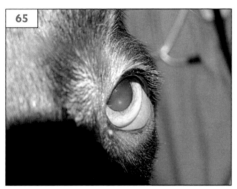

65 Chemosis in a patient with hypoproteinemia and interstitial fluid volume overload.

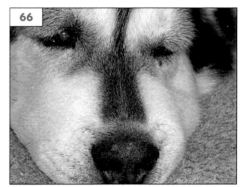

66 An Alaskan malamute with severe peripheral edema from vasculitis and systemic inflammatory response syndrome secondary to severe pancreatitis. In this case, vasculitis combined with a decrease in colloid oncotic pressure and interstitial crystalloid fluid overload contributed to significant peripheral edema.

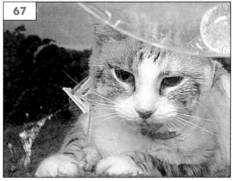

67 Pulmonary edema fluid in a cat with congestive heart failure.

Central venous pressure monitoring

The central venous pressure (CVP) is an indirect measurement of intravascular fluid volume. More accurately, the CVP is a measure of the hydrostatic pressure in the cranial vena cava just outside the right atrium in the absence of veno-occlusive disease.[10] Other factors that influence an animal's CVP include vasomotor tone, right heart function, intrathoracic pressure, and vascular compliance.[10] The CVP can be measured directly using a pressure-transducer connected to a central venous catheter whose tip is located just outside the right atrium. If a CVP transducer is not available, the CVP can be measured using lengths of intravenous extension tubing and a water manometer. In large dogs, the most accurate measurement of CVP is obtained with a jugular central venous catheter whose tip is located just outside the right atrium (**68**). In cats and puppies, however, trends of CVP can be accurately assessed with a central venous catheter placed in the jugular vein, or in the lateral or medial saphenous veins such that the catheter tip is located in the caudal vena cava (**69**). [15,16]

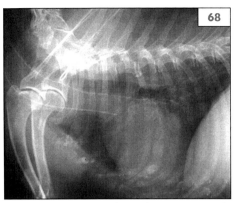

68 Lateral thoracic radiograph in a patient with a long catheter in the jugular vein. Note that with the tip of the catheter at or near the right atrium, the catheter can be used to measure central venous pressure.

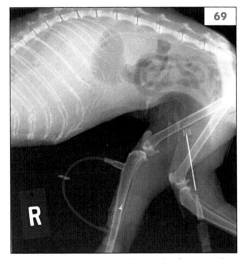

69 Lateral abdominal radiograph of a cat with a central catheter placed into the medial saphenous vein. The tip of the catheter is in the caudal vena cava, and can be used to measure central venous pressure if desired.

A three-way stop-cock has two female ports and one male port. To measure the CVP, a length of IV extension tubing is secured to one of the female ports of a three-way stop-cock. A 20–35 mL syringe of heparinized 0.9% sterile saline is then connected to the other female port of the stop-cock. A water manometer should be connected to the third port of the stop-cock (**70**). The stop-cock should be turned to allow flushing of the length of IV extensions tubing with the heparinized saline (**71**). Next, the male port of the extension tubing should be connected to the female port of the central venous catheter. The stop-cock is closed so that the fluid is 'off' to the patient, to allow the fluid column in the water manometer to fill (**72**), taking care to avoid introducing air bubbles into the water column that can interfere with accurate CVP measurement. Once the fluid column is >20 cmH$_2$O, the zero mark on the water manometer is held adjacent to the manubrium of the animal (this approximates the catheter tip near the right heart), and the stop-cock is

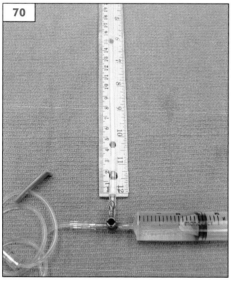

70 In addition to placement of a long central venous catheter, supplies required for measurement of central venous pressure include a 20 or 30 mL syringe with sterile 0.9% saline, lengths of IV extension tubing, and a water or column manometer. If a manometer is not available, a length of IV extension tubing taped to a metric ruler with gradations in centimeters can be used in its place, and is less costly.

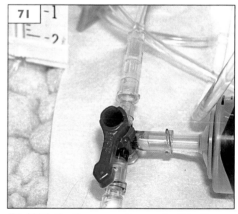

71 With the three-way stop-cock off to the patient, saline is pushed into the manometer. Take care to not introduce air bubbles in the manometer. The stop-cock should be turned to allow flushing of the length of IV extension tubing with the heparinized saline.

turned 'off' to the syringe (73). This will create a fluid column between the manometer and the patient. The fluid column will slowly drop until the meniscus stabilizes and then rises and falls with the animal's heartbeat and respiration. It is at this point that the value adjacent to the lower portion of the meniscus is read to indicate CVP. Several measurements should be obtained, throwing out any values that may be artifactually high or low. It is important to remember to record exactly where the zero mark on the manometer was used to measure the CVP, to avoid conflicting results when measurements are obtained by different personnel in the same animal.

Normal CVP values are 0–5 cmH_2O in healthy euvolemic animals. Lower CVP measurements (i.e. <0 cmH_2O) are usually indicative of a decrease in intravascular fluid volume, or may be secondary to vasodilation.[10] CVP values greater than 10–12 cmH_2O are usually indicative of a greater risk of intravascular volume overload, or may be observed with significant quantities of pleural

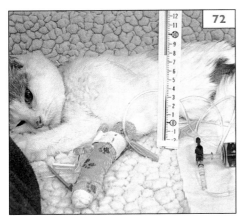

72 Cat with a jugular and a cephalic catheter in place. The zero mark on the manometer (note that in this case, the manometer is a length of IV extension tubing and a metric ruler) is placed at the level of the cat's manubrium, or sternum, such that it is at the level of the right atrium.

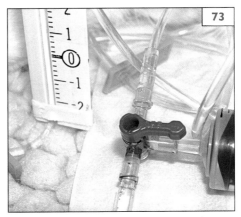

73 With the three-way stop-cock closed to the syringe, and the zero point on the manometer at the level of the cat's right atrium, the fluid column is allowed to equilibrate. Once the fluid column moves up and down with the patient's heartbeat, the lowest point of the meniscus can be measured as the central venous pressure in centimeters of water (cmH_2O).

effusion and/or right-sided heart failure.[10] Ideally, the animal's CVP should be 7–10 cmH_2O (*Table 13*). In some animals the baseline CVP measurement may be greater than 10 cmH_2O due to kinks in the catheter or improper catheter placement, or due to increased circulating intravascular fluid. In such animals, if intravenous fluid therapy is necessary, the CVP should not increase by more than 5 cmH_2O in any 24 hour period. If there is an inherent risk of intravascular volume overload, other additional parameters should be closely monitored, including respiratory rate and effort, thoracic auscultation for pulmonary crackles, serous nasal discharge, or chemosis. If such clinical signs occur, intravenous fluids should be reduced or stopped, and a diuretic can be administered.

Table 13
Measurement and interpretation of central venous pressure

Central venous pressure (cmH_2O)	Interpretation	Possible cause(s)
<2	Severe hypovolemia	Severe intravascular fluid volume deficit
		Severe dehydration
		Inaccurate measurement
		Vasodilation
–2 to 0	Hypovolemia	intravascular fluid volume deficit
		Vasodilation
		Inaccurate measurement
0 – 5	Euvolemia	Normal intravascular volume status
		Normal right heart function
5 to 10	Normal to slight increase in CVP	May be normal
		Increased intravascular fluid volume status
		Decreased inflow into right heart (myocardial disease, heartbase tumor, pericardial effusion)
		Inaccurate measurement
		Possible impending fluid volume overload, use caution
> 10	Increased CVP	Increased intravascular volume status
		Kinked catheter
		Decreased inflow into right heart (myocardial disease, heartbase tumor, pericardial tamponade)
		Inaccurate measurement
		Impending intravascular fluid volume overload

Electrolyte derangements secondary to crystalloid fluid administration

There is a huge variety of crystalloid fluids that can be used in small animal patients. The intravenous fluid chosen should ideally be based on a patient's acid–base and electrolyte status. For example, in an animal with a hypochloremic metabolic alkalosis due to a pyloric outflow obstruction, administration of a fluid that contains buffers may academically be inappropriate when other more acidifying solutions with a higher chloride content are available, such as 0.9% sodium chloride. The administration of 0.9% sodium chloride can, however, potentially exacerbate hypernatremia or hyperchloremia, and should be used with caution in a patient with such metabolic derangements. In an animal with metabolic acidosis, the administration of an acidifying solution that contains no buffers, such as 0.9% sodium chloride or 5DW, can potentially worsen the metabolic acidosis, or at best delay the correction of the low pH. In cases of metabolic acidosis due to severe hypoperfusion and impaired oxygen delivery, the administration of any isotonic crystalloid fluid, even those without any buffers, can help to restore perfusion and improve oxygen delivery and correct lactic acidosis once intravascular fluid volume is restored.

Lactated Ringer's solution contains a small amount of calcium. This may potentially be beneficial in an animal with hypocalcemia, such as a bitch with eclampsia, for example, but could be inappropriate for an animal with hypercalcemia secondary to a malignancy or hyperparathyroidism. Similarly, administering a fluid that contains potassium to an animal with hypokalemia is beneficial, but potentially can be detrimental for an animal with severe hyperkalemia. In general, the administration of intravenous fluids to an animal with intravascular volume depletion and dehydration can restore intravascular and interstitial volume, and can dilute serum electrolyte concentrations. Restoration of intravascular fluid volume also commonly helps to correct acid–base abnormalities such as a metabolic acidosis, and the correction can also improve hyperkalemia as potassium is exchanged for hydrogen by the sodium–potassium–ATPase pump.

Overzealous rapid administration of hypotonic solutions such as 5DW can potentially lead to intravascular hemolysis, and can promote hyperglycemia. At slower infusion rates the dextrose in D5W is metabolized quickly, and essentially infuses free water without causing intravascular hemolysis. The administration of large volumes of dextrose-containing fluids can cause hyperglycemia and potentially cerebral edema, which can worsen the prognosis in animals with traumatic brain injury.[17] Rapid administration of hypertonic saline can result in damage to red blood cells and crenation.[13] Rapid infusion of hypertonic saline can also cause hypotension and bradycardia due to vagal stimulation, and should not be administered to patients that are severely dehydrated or hypernatremic.[3] Administration of a calcium-containing fluid in the same line as blood products can cause the precipitation of calcium citrate, and should be avoided.

CHAPTER 4

Colloids

- **Introduction**

- **Colloid characteristics**

- **Colloids**

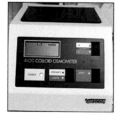 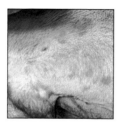 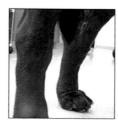

INTRODUCTION

A colloid fluid contains large molecular weight particles. The semipermeable membrane of the healthy vasculature is relatively impermeable to such particles. The number of particles in the colloid solution promotes the retention of sodium and water around the core of the particle within the vascular space. Depending on the colloid oncotic pressure of the solution (COP), some colloid solutions can also draw fluid into the intravascular space from other fluid compartments in the body.[1] Colloid fluids can be categorized as either natural or synthetic. Natural colloids include whole blood with plasma proteins, plasma, and concentrated albumin solutions.[2] Synthetic colloids include dextran-70, oxypolygelatin, hydroxyethyl starch, and pentastarch. Colloid solutions are useful during the treatment of conditions associated with hypovolemic and septic shock, vasculitis, hypoproteinemia, and third-spacing of fluids such as pleural and peritoneal effusions and peripheral edema.[1]

COLLOID CHARACTERISTICS

Colloid oncotic pressure

Fluid movement between compartments is regulated by the relative balance of COP and hydrostatic pressure on either side of the vasculature's semipermeable membrane (**74**). Other factors that can also influence the movement or retention of a particle within the vascular space and interstitium are the particle size, the pore size of the vasculature, and the charge of the particle. The COP is the force exerted by the size and number of large molecular weight molecules on either side of a semipermeable membrane. The plasma proteins albumin, globulin, and fibrinogen contribute to the COP of the intravascular space.[3] Of these proteins, albumin contributes approximately 75–80% to the COP, whereas globulin proteins contribute 20–25% to the COP.[3] A normal COP in dogs is 19.95 ± 2.1 mmHg, and in cats is 24.7 ± 3.7 mmHg.[4,5] If an animal's COP is less than 14 mmHg, the patient is at significant risk of developing interstitial edema.[6] The goal or end-point of colloid fluid administration should be to produce a COP of 14–18 mmHg.[6] Because the duration of the sustained effect of each colloid varies, it is generally recommended that with any colloid infusion, the infusion should be continued until the animal is able to maintain its serum COP without additional support.

As discussed in Chapter 1, hydrostatic pressure is the force exerted by water molecules within the different fluid compartments. A massive infusion of a crystalloid fluid effectively increases the hydrostatic pressure within the intravascular fluid compartment and dilutes the colloid molecules within that compartment, such that intravascular hydrostatic forces increase and allow movement of the fluid from the intravascular space into the interstitium. Infusion of a natural or synthetic colloid, however, will increase the COP within the intravascular compartment in relation to the interstitial compartment.

Infusion of colloid fluids that contain relatively larger numbers of smaller particles will cause an initial increase in serum oncotic pressure. Smaller particles are degraded more quickly, and the larger particles are responsible

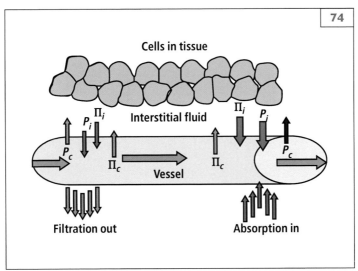

74 Starling's forces govern the fluid flux, or movement of fluid, between compartments, namely, the interstitial and intravascular spaces. Fluid flux is dependent on the pressure gradients of the oncotic forces (Π) and hydrostatic forces (P) in between the interstitial and intravascular fluid spaces, the capillary pore size, and the filtration coefficient.

for the sustained effect or the longevity of the colloid in the vascular space.[2] As long as the vasculature is healthy and remains impermeable to the large molecular weight particles, the particles can exert a water-attracting force within the intravascular fluid compartment. By increasing the number of colloid particles that retain water within the vasculature, the effective water-holding capacity of the intravascular space is increased. Following the infusion of a colloid, fluid can be drawn into the intravascular compartment from the interstitium. In most instances, however, concurrent administration of a colloid solution simultaneously with a crystalloid solution will favor the intravascular retention of water from the crystalloid fluid infused for a longer period of time than if the crystalloid solution was infused alone.

Without a colloid, approximately 80% of a crystalloid fluid infused will leave the intravascular space within 1 hour of administration. With concurrent administration of a colloid, the crystalloid fluid will be retained within the vascular space for a longer period. This can potentially increase the capillary hydrostatic pressure and lead to interstitial, including pulmonary, edema. To avoid this potential complication, the crystalloid fluid volume should be reduced by 25–50% when a colloid is infused concurrently. That is, only 50–75% of the calculated crystalloid fluid volume should be administered to avoid the potential for interstitial edema. Both clinically and experimentally, an increase in intravascular lung water during resuscitation from hemorrhagic shock can reduce serum COP and reduce oxygen delivery.[7,8]

The Gibbs–Donnan effect

Proteins in solution carry a net negative charge. Positively charged ions such as sodium are attracted around the protein's core structure to balance the charge towards electrical neutrality.[3] When a colloid is infused into the bloodstream, water follows sodium and is attracted to the core structure of the protein molecule, causing the water to remain within the intravascular space (**75**).

Because of the water-attracting property of the negatively charged colloid particles in solution, the COP of plasma is greater than what would be expected based on the presence and osmotic pressure of the proteins alone (**76**).[3]

Colloid osmometry

The Landis–Pappenheimer equation can be used to estimate the plasma COP based on an animal's total protein (TPr):

$$COP \ (mmHg) = 2.1(TPr) + 0.16(TPr^2) + (TPr^3)$$

This equation is not very sensitive or accurate in critically ill animals because of changes in serum pH, acid–base status, albumin: globulin ratios, and the concurrent administration of synthetic colloids.[9–11]

A colloid osmometer is an instrument that measures the COP of a fluid.[6] The Wescor 4420 colloid osmometer (**77**) has a pressure transducer that senses the pressure difference between a chamber filled with saline and a chamber filled with blood or plasma. A net flux of fluid occurs from the test chamber into the patient's sample chamber owing to differences in the osmolality of the fluids within each chamber. The pressure gradient that is generated is recorded in mmHg.[6] If a colloid osmometer is not available, plasma albumin concentration and total solids can be used as a rough indicator to assess the need for colloid therapy. Albumin contributes roughly 50% to the plasma total solids, if hyperglobulinemia is not present. If total solids are less than 4.0 g/dL (40 g/L), or albumin is less than 2 g/dL (20 g/L), oncotic support is necessary.

75 A colloid solution contains large molecular weight particles that are osmotically active and draw sodium around their core structures. Wherever sodium is, water follows. By attracting sodium and water around the particle, water is held within the vascular space.[3,6]

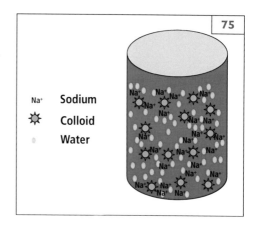

Na⁺   Sodium

☼   Colloid

○   Water

76 Colloid oncotic pressure and the Gibbs–Donnan effect. Normal serum oncotic pressure ranges from 17 to 22 mmHg. When the colloid oncotic pressure (COP) of a fluid is supraphysiologic and exceeds the patient's normal COP, infusion of the colloid into the intravascular space will draw fluid from the interstitium. The fluid expansion property of a fluid that exceeds what is expected from the colloid alone is known as the Gibbs–Donnan effect, and is caused by the attraction of positive ions such as sodium and water around the negative core structure of the colloid.[3,6]

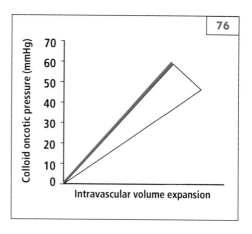

77 Wescor 4420 colloid osmometer.

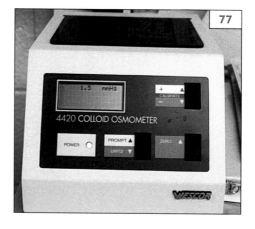

Table 14
Conditions that can cause vasculitis and increased capillary pore size

Decreased albumin production
    Hepatic failure
    Starvation
    Malnutrition
    Excessive colloid administration
Increased protein loss
    Protein-losing nephropathy
    Protein-losing enteropathy
        Inflammatory bowel disease
        Lymphangectasia
        Neoplasia
    Third-spacing of fluids
        Peritonitis
            Feline Infectious Peritonitis (FIP)
            Sepsis
            Pancreatitis
        Pleural effusions
            FIP
            Chylothorax
            Pyothorax
        Trauma
            Shearing injury
            Burns
Vasculitis
        Parvoviral enteritis
        Pancreatitis
        Pyometra
        Immune-mediated vasculitis
        Heat-induced illness
        Snake envenomation
        Burns
        Neoplasia
        Crush injury
        Trauma

Hypoalbuminemia can be associated with decreased production due to hepatic failure or severe starvation; however, in the majority of cases, hypoalbuminemia is caused by increased loss due to infectious, inflammatory, or immune-mediated diseases.

Indications for colloids

Approximately 75–80% of an isotonic crystalloid fluid infused will leave the intravascular space within 1 hour of infusion.[5] Infusion of a colloid fluid along with a crystalloid fluid will help retain the fluid within the vascular space for a longer period of time and have a sustained effect on intravascular volume expansion. For this reason, colloid infusions are often administered in combination with a crystalloid fluid during hypovolemic shock. Fluid is also retained within the intravascular space as a result of the net effect of the difference between oncotic and hydrostatic pressures within the intravascular and interstitial fluid compartments. An important factor in fluid retention is also the pore size of the vasculature. Any condition that is associated with sepsis, vasculitis, or systemic inflammatory response syndrome can predispose the leakage of intravascular fluid into the interstitium (*Table 14*). Additionally, conditions that are associated with hypoalbuminemia (albumin <2.0 g/dL [20 g/L]) can result in decreased intravascular COP to such an extent that capillary hydrostatic pressures predominate in favoring the efflux of intravascular fluid into the interstitium. Under normal circumstances, lymphatic drainage picks up excessive interstitial fluid and transports it back into the vasculature. In situations associated with increased intravascular hydrostatic pressure or decreased oncotic pressure, or with increased capillary pore size, lymphatic drainage can become overwhelmed and lead to interstitial edema.

Potential complications of colloids

The use of colloid fluids should not be viewed as failsafe or innocuous, and they should always be used with caution. One must consider the potential risks when determining whether a patient will benefit from administration of a natural or synthetic colloid solution. The benefits of colloids are that they can help restore intravascular fluid volume, systemic blood pressure, and perfusion and oxygen delivery to vital organs during the treatment of hypovolemic shock and third-spacing of fluids. Because colloid-containing fluids exert a moderate to potent attraction of water into the intravascular space, they can potentially contribute to intravascular volume overload in predisposed patients, or to congestive heart failure in patients with an even mild to moderate degree of cardiac dysfunction. Any animal with a potential for intravascular volume overload should be monitored carefully for clinical signs of chemosis, increased respiratory rate and effort, pulmonary crackles, serous nasal discharge, and subcutaneous edema. Ideally, colloid support should be titrated based on changes in the animal's COP measured by a colloid osmometer.[6] Realistically, colloid osmometry is not available in all veterinary practices. When a colloid osmometer is unavailable, total solids or plasma albumin concentration can also be used as a rough guide as to when colloid support is necessary. In such instances, therapy with crystalloid and colloid fluids should be titrated based on changes in the animal's body weight, CVP, and response of perfusion parameters with therapy. Specific potential complications associated with each colloid will be discussed in detail separately.

COLLOIDS

Properties and recommended doses of colloids for use in veterinary patients are listed in *Tables 15* and *16*.

Hydroxyethyl starch (hetastarch) solutions contain a synthetic polymer of amylopectin, a highly branched starch molecule in 0.9% saline or lactated Ringer's solution (*Table 15*). The branched nature of the polymer produces a fluid that contains molecules of various sizes that range from 10,000 to 10^6 Daltons (Da). The average weight of the solution is 69,000–71,000 Da, a molecule that is very similar in size to naturally occurring serum albumin.[1] Approximately one-third of hetastarch remains in circulation after 3 days, and can be detected in serum for up to 17 weeks in humans.[12] Smaller particles (<50,000 Da) are degraded by serum amylase and excreted by the kidneys. Larger molecules are metabolized by the reticuloendothelial system. In dogs, the half-life is shorter, at 7–9 days. Approximately 30% is degraded and eliminated within 24 hours.[13-15] In dogs and cats, published recommended doses of hetastarch are 20–30 mL/kg/day because of the potential risks of coagulopathy as the amylopectin polymer binds with von

Table 15
Properties of colloid solutions

Colloid fluid	Colloid oncotic pressure (mmHg)	Serum half-life	Intravascular volume expansion	Average molecular weight (Daltons)
25% Albumin	70	16 hr	4–5	69,000
6% Dextran-70	60	7–9 hr	0.8	41,000
Oxypolygelatin (Vetaplasma)	46	2 hr	1.0	35,000
10% Dextran-40	40	30 min	1–1.5	26,000
Voluven (6% hydroxyethyl starch 130/0.4 in 0.9% NaCl)	36	4–6 hr	1	130,000
6% Hydroxyethyl starch	35	7–9 days	1–1.3	69,000
10% Pentastarch	32	10 hr	1.5	120,000
5% Albumin	20	16 hr	0.7–1.3	69,000

Colloid fluids that have an oncotic pressure similar to that of plasma possess a lower capacity for intravascular volume expansion than fluids such as 25% albumin. Hydroxyethyl starch has a similar average molecular weight to albumin, the protein found naturally within the body that contributes 75–80% to the colloid oncotic pressure of plasma.

Willebrand factor. In practice, however, this recommended dose can be exceeded when hetastarch solutions are being used to improve blood pressure. The colloid infusion can be administered in 5–10 mL/kg increments when attempting to improve hypotension, and then continued as a constant-rate infusion when using it to contribute to colloid oncotic pressure (*Table 16*). In animals with low oncotic pressure, or hypoalbuminemia, supplemental colloid support should be continued until the source of albumin loss and clinical signs attributable to hypoalbuminemia (i.e. chemosis, pulmonary edema, peripheral edema) have resolved.

Pentastarch is also known as low-molecular weight hetastarch. Pentastarch also contains polymers of amylopectin, with a more homogeneous and average molecular weight of 30,000 Da.[2] Pentastarch provides a rapid increase in blood volume within 1 hour of administration.[2] Because of the smaller size of the majority of pentastarch particles, the elimination half-life is more rapid than that of hetastarch. Approximately 90% of pentastarch is cleared from the circulation within 24 hours of administration, and the rest is gone after 3 days.[12]

Table 16
Recommended doses of colloid solutions available for use in veterinary patients

Colloid	Recommended bolus dose (mL) dogs	Recommended bolus dose (mL) cats	Recommended daily dose (CRI mL/kg/day) dogs	Recommended daily dose (CRI mL/kg/day) cats
Hydroxyethyl starch	5–10 mL/kg	5 mL/kg	20–30 mL/kg/day	20 mL/kg/day
Dextran-70	5–10 mL/kg	5 mL/kg	20–30 mL/kg/day	20 mL/kg/day
Pentastarch	10–40 mL/kg	5 mL/kg	10–25 mL/kg/day	5–10 mL/kg/day
25% albumin	4–5 mL/kg to treat hypotension	2–3 mL/kg to treat hypotension	5 mL/kg/day total dose, although may need to go higher with ongoing losses	3 mL/kg/day total dose, although may need to go higher with ongoing losses
Oxypolygelatin	3–5 mL/kg over 15 min, then 5–15 mL/kg more slowly	3–5 mL/kg over 15 min, then 5–15 mL/kg slowly	20 mL/kg/day	20 mL/kg/day

The amylopectin in both hetastarch and pentastarch solutions is degraded by serum amylase, and as such can result in a mild increase in serum amylase concentration. By no means should this be interpreted as a cause and effect of hetastarch causing pancreatitis, as serum amylase concentration is a very insensitive clinical marker for this disease. Hetastarch can decrease Von Willebrand factor and factor VII activities to 40% of normal.[16] Monitoring of the intrinsic clotting cascade, that is, the activated clotting time (ACT) and activated partial thromboplastin time (APTT), may show elevations above normal reference values in animals that have received hetastarch.[17] Platelet plug formation may also be delayed in dogs after administration of various hetastarch solutions.[18] This is likely not clinically significant and does not cause clinical bleeding until the infusion exceeds the manufacturer's recommended dose of no more than 20–30 mL/kg/day, or if an animal has a hereditary coagulation disorder such as a factor VII deficiency or von Willebrand's disease.[16,17,19] When administered too rapidly, hetastarch can cause histamine release in cats, and has been known to cause vomiting.[2,5] Because of this effect, it is generally recommended to avoid rapid boluses of the solutions over less than 15 minutes in this species.

Dextran-40 and Dextran-70

Dextran-containing solutions have been used for decades to provide colloidal support, although these solutions are not widely used in current practice. Dextran solutions are essentially polymers of glucose produced by a bacterium (*Leuconostoc mesenteroides*).[1] Dextran-40 contains glucose polymers with an average molecular weight of 40,000 Da, and Dextran-70 contains glucose polymers with an average molecular weight of 70,000 Da. The half-lives of the above solutions are approximately 30 minutes and 7–9 hours, respectively (*Table 15*).

The administration of Dextran-containing fluids is not innocuous. Dextrans are excreted by the kidneys. Half-lives can be greatly prolonged in animals with renal insufficiency and decreased glomerular clearance.[1] In addition, low-volume or hypotensive states can reduce or prolong renal clearance and cause precipitation of the polymer in the renal tubules. This can potentially lead to renal failure.[20] For this reason, Dextran-containing fluids should be used with caution in hypovolemic, hypotensive, dehydrated patients, and those with renal dysfunction.[1] Dextran-70 can promote neutrophil demargination and reduce neutrophil counts in animals.[21] Dextrans can coat red blood cells and platelets, and interfere with tests of coagulation and red cell cross-match procedures.

Humans and some small animals possess naturally occurring antibodies against the Dextran molecule. These are thought to develop from exposure to Dextran-containing foodstuffs. Rapid infusion of Dextrans, particularly Dextran-40, have been associated with anaphylactic reactions. For this reason, the use of Dextran-40 has largely fallen out of favor in both humans and veterinary patients. Dextran-70 can coat platelets and reduce aggregability, and can prolong bleeding times. This may be beneficial in hypercoagulable states such as that observed with hyperadrenocorticism or Disseminated Intravascular Coagulation (DIC), but would largely be contraindicated in animals with thrombocytopenia or thrombocytopathia. Additionally, refractometric readings of COP can be artifactually reduced by the dilutional effects of hetastarch or Dextrans.[4]

Oxypolygelatin

Gelatin solutions were initially developed for use in mass casualty situations, and are widely available in Europe. Gelatin solutions contain modified and urea cross-linked gelatin of bovine collagen origin.[1] The average molecular weight of the particles in solution is approximately 30,000–35,000 Da. Because of the large number and small size of the particles in solution, oxypolygelatin acts as a potent colloid and draws a volume of fluid from the interstitial space into the vasculature equal to the amount administered. Oxypolygelatin has a relatively short half-life of 2 hours (*Table 15*),[1] but can be found in the circulation for approximately 7 days after administration. Like other synthetic colloids, oxypolygelatin is excreted by the kidneys and should be used with caution in animals with renal insufficiency or failure. The risk of anaphylaxis is low[7], but it can occur.[1,5] Although oxypolygelatin has not been shown to affect platelets or clotting factor proteins, dilutional coagulopathies can occur after administration of large volumes.[1,5]

Concentrated human albumin

Concentrated human and canine-specific albumin solutions are now available for use in veterinary patients. During states of health, albumin contributes approximately 50% to the serum total protein and 80% to the serum COP.[11] Extrapolation of COP from serum albumin has been reported, but is largely inaccurate in animals.[9–11] Therefore, use of a colloid osmometer is considered the gold standard if an animal is at risk of developing interstitial edema secondary to hypo-albuminemia. The majority of albumin within the body is located in the interstitial compartment, with a smaller amount located intravascularly. This becomes important in disease states associated with hypoalbuminemia. In such instances, the intravascular pool becomes replenished by the interstitial pool and hepatic synthesis until this supply becomes depleted. Albumin synthesis by the liver is stimulated by osmoreceptors in the hepatic sinusoids sensing a decrease in COP. In the presence of synthetic colloids, the osmoreceptors sense an artifactual increase to normal COP at the hepatic sinusoid, and albumin production may be curtailed. Once significant hypoalbuminemia (albumin <2.0 g/dL [20 g/L]) develops, the intravascular hydrostatic pressure can exceed intravascular COP, and lead to efflux of fluid from the intravascular space into the interstitium, overwhelming the lymphatic drainage system and leading to interstitial edema. Hypoalbuminemia with serum albumin <2.0 g/dL (20 g/L) has been associated with a significantly increased risk of mortality in critically ill dogs,[22] enteral feeding intolerance, and delayed wound healing.[23]

In addition to contributing the majority of the COP in the body, albumin also has important functions as a mediator of coagulation, drug and hormone carrier, scavenger of oxygen-derived free-radical

species, and mediator of healing.[24] In both human and animal patients with clinically significant hypoalbuminemia, morbidity and mortality are increased unless albumin stores are replenished.[22–24] Plasma solutions contain small amounts of albumin, but are an inefficient and costly means of replenishing serum and interstitial albumin concentrations.[24] To raise the serum albumin by 0.5 g/dL (5 g/L) in a hypoalbuminemic animal, approximately 20 mL/kg of plasma must be administered. This dose increases if ongoing albumin losses are present.

Most recently, concentrated human albumin solutions have been used for a number of reasons, including treatment of hypoalbuminemia and decreased COP, and as a potent colloid in the treatment of hypotension (*Table 17*).[25,26]

Table 17

Recommendations for administration of concentrated (25%) human albumin[25]

(1) Test dose 0.25 mL/kg/hr for 15 minutes

(2) Watch for clinical signs of albumin reaction:

    Facial swelling/angioneurotic edema

    Urticaria

    Hypotension

    Vomiting

    Tachycardia

    Tachypnea

    Fever

(3) Administer as a constant rate infusion:

    Slow bolus 2–4 mL/kg to treat hypotension or

    5 mL/kg slowly or

    0.1–1.7 mL/kg/hr over 4–8 hours

(4) Refrigerate and use remainder within 24 hours or discard

Medical therapy with a combination of fresh frozen plasma or concentrated 25% human albumin to increase serum albumin to 2.0 g/dL (20 g/L) can greatly improve clinical outcome. To calculate the albumin deficit:

Albumin deficit = 10 × (desired [albumin]g/dL – patient [albumin]g/dL) × BW$_{kg}$ × 0.3.[27]

Processed canine plasma typically contains 20–30 g/L of albumin. When using this formula to determine the albumin deficit, it quickly becomes obvious that administration of plasma to replenish albumin is often cost-prohibitive.

Both immediate and delayed rare hypersensitivity reactions have occurred in critically ill dogs, and include fever, vomiting, angioneurotic edema, delayed vasculitis, and polyarthopathies.[28–30] A prospective study documented a high rate of development of antialbumin antibodies and complications when concentrated human albumin was infused into healthy, normoalbuminemic dogs.[28,29] A limitation of this study was that all experimental dogs were normoalbuminemic and received a very large dose (50 g) of human albumin within 1 hour, rather than the recommended smaller dose and slower rate over 4–8 hours. The authors acknowledged that immunocompetence in normoalbuminemic dogs differs from that in critically ill animals, and may put the normoalbuminemic animals at a particular risk of developing antihuman albumin antibodies and reactions to albumin infusion.[28] In a later study, the researchers documented that all dogs, both experimental and clinical cases, that received human albumin developed antialbumin antibodies within days to weeks after infusion.[29] Early reactions occurred during albumin infusion, while delayed reactions occurred approximately 6–14 days later. Two healthy dogs that received concentrated human albumin developed vasculitis after administration, and then died.

Clients must be made aware of the potential risks of complications. However, two studies have documented marked benefit and improved survival in animals that were poorly responsive to other more conventional therapies in the intensive care units.[25,26] Because of the inherent risks associated with the administration of concentrated human albumin to dogs, its infusion should be restricted to animals with acute severe hypoalbuminemia whose clinical signs and conditions are not sufficiently treated with blood products and artificial colloids alone. In general, once serum albumin has increased to 2.0 g/dL (20 g/L), COP can be maintained through use of a synthetic colloid such as hetastarch, pentastarch, voluven, or Dextran-70.

This author has used concentrated human albumin (25%) with success and minimal adverse reactions in clinical practice in severely hypoalbuminemic dogs; however, the potential benefits associated with its use must be considered and outweigh potential risks on a case-by-case basis (**78, 79**).

Canine-specific albumin has been purified by Animal Blood Resources International. The product is available as 5 g vials. For hypovolemic shock, a dose of 1 mL/minute of the 16%, not to exceed 2.5–5 mL/kg/day. To correct hypoalbuminemia, the recommended dose is 5–6 mL/kg of the 16% solution, not to exceed 2 g/kg of albumin per day. The half-life of canine-specific purified albumin is 12–15 days, and it is eliminated from circulation in 20–24 days. As with all other blood products, canine-specific albumin must be used within 24 hours, then discarded, because of the potential for bacterial growth and infection.

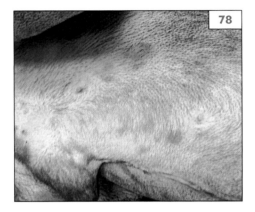

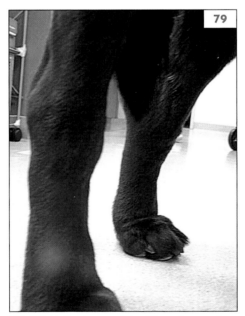

78, 79 Urticaria, vasculitis pitting edema and joint effusion in a dog 2 weeks after administration of 25% concentrated human albumin.

Canine and feline blood banking and blood product administration

- **Introduction**
- **Economics of blood banking**
- **Selection of donors**
- **Blood typing**
- **Cross-match procedure**
- **Blood collection**
- **Blood components**
- **Transfusion therapy**

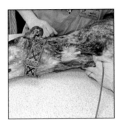
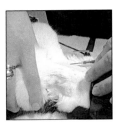
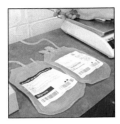
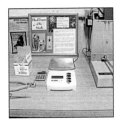

INTRODUCTION

Many centuries ago, the concept of 'like transfuses like' was discovered when infusion of blood from one species into a different species was met with ultimately fatal complications. In the early 1600s, Richard Lower withdrew blood from the femoral artery of one dog, then infused it into the jugular vein of another dog, without complications.[1] However, infusion of sheep and cow blood into humans resulted in fever, nausea, renal pain, and black discoloration of the urine. In 1910, four different agglutinins and hemolysins on canine red blood cells were discovered.[1] Since that time, a total of 12 canine erythrocyte antigen (DEA) blood groups have been discovered in dogs, and four different blood types in domestic cats,[2] and veterinarians now have a much more solid working knowledge of transfusion medicine for small animal patients. Administration of whole blood and specific blood components has become a mainstay in the therapy of critically ill patients with various forms of anemia and abnormalities of coagulation. A thorough knowledge of the components of each blood product, indications for its use, and potential risks of administration are necessary to provide appropriate therapies for the patient, and to make the most of blood banks and donor pools.

ECONOMICS OF BLOOD BANKING

When considering whether to start a blood bank at a small animal practice, the practitioner must evaluate a number of factors practically, economically, and ethically. Consider the frequency with which blood products are needed at the facility. Is it hardly ever, once or twice a month, or almost every day? If the first, then the economics of keeping a closed colony of donor dogs and cats is wasteful. If the use of blood products is regular but still fairly infrequent, purchase and storage of the blood products is likely to be more cost-effective than housing donors. Even with extremely frequent use, it is very difficult to make a blood banking service a profitable business, as the products themselves cannot be cost-prohibitive for the client to purchase for their animal's treatment. There are numerous expenses involved in maintaining a donor colony, including technician time, purchase and maintenance of a refrigerated centrifuge, screening for underlying illness and potential infectious diseases, a plasma extractor, as well as refrigeration and freezer units for blood product storage. Other costs include the cost of daily care, housing, feeding, and medical care of the donor animals. Finally, and very importantly, one must consider the animal's quality of life at the hospital. A viable alternative to minimizing the above expenses and providing a good quality of life for the donor animals is to have an out-of-hospital donor pool with scheduled collection dates to keep up with the hospital's needs. In practice, this works well, and the animals have a greater quality of life than living at an animal hospital.

SELECTION OF DONORS

Canine donors

The ideal canine donor should have a friendly yet calm temperament and should not become stressed during collection. Blood donors should receive annual physical examinations and general health screens, including a complete blood count, serum biochemistry panel, and occult heartworm antigen test.[3] A consensus panel of the American College of Veterinary Internal Medicine suggested various categories of conditional testing and mandatory testing for vector-borne and nonvector-borne diseases (*Table 18*).[4] Organisms that can be transmitted to recipients from donor blood, can cause subclinical infection in a donor, can be cultured from the blood of an infected animal, or can result in a significant difficult to treat infection should be tested for in all canine and feline donors. Canine donors should also be screened initially for *Babesia canis* and *B. gibsoni*, *Leishmania donovani*, *Ehrlichia canis*, and brucellosis (*Brucella canis*). Other conditionally recommended tests include for anaplasmosis (*Anaplasma phagocytophilum* and *A. platys*), neorickettsiosis (*Neorickettsia risticii* and *N. helmintheca*), *Mycoplasma haemocanis* (*Hemobartonella canis*), hemoplasmosis, and in dogs from Texas or the southwest United States, *Trypanosoma cruzi*, or Chagas' disease. Routine testing for *Rickettsia rickettsii* (Rocky Mountain spotted fever) or *Borrelia burgdorferi* (Lyme disease) is not recommended. There have been documented reports of donor blood causing babesiosis and leishmaniasis in recipient dogs.[5,6] Dogs should ideally weigh more than 50 lb (27 kg), be between 1 and 8 years of age, have a packed cell volume (PCV) of at least 40%, be spayed or neutered, and have never received a transfusion.

Table 18
Recommended screening tests for canine blood donors (adapted from ACVIM Consensus Statement)[4]

Disease	Infective organism	Test
Babesiosis	*Babesia canis*	IFA or PCR
	Babesia gibsoni	IFA or PCR
Ehrlichiosis	*Ehrlichia canis*	IFA, PCR,
		or ELISA
Brucellosis	*Brucella canis*	RSAT or
		TAT
Leishmaniasis	*Leishmania donovani*	IFA or PCR

ELISA: enzyme-linked immunosorbent assay; IFA: immunofluorescent assay; PCR: polymerase chain reaction; RSAT: rapid slide agglutination test; TAT: tube agglutination test.

Feline donors

Like the canine donor, the feline donor should have a good temperament and not be stressed during physical examination. Due to the inherent nature of the cat's smaller body and vein size, many donors must be placed under extremely heavy sedation or general anesthesia for sample collection. Feline blood donors should ideally weigh more than 10 lb (4.5 kg), be between 1 and 8 years of age, be spayed or neutered, and have never received a transfusion.[4] Additionally, donor cats should be screened for feline leukemia virus (FeLV), feline immunodeficiency virus (FIV), hemoplasmosis (*Mycoplasma haemofelis* and *M. haemominutum*), and bartonellosis (*Bartonella henselae*, *B. clarridgeae* and *B. kholerae*) prior to donation (*Table 19*). Testing for *Cytauxzoon felis*, ehrlichiosis, anaplasmosis, and neorickettsia is not routinely recommended in cats. Because feline infectious peritonitis (FIP) testing is often equivocal in cats, routine antibody titers to coronavirus are not recommended. Further routine screening for *Toxoplasma gondii* is also not routinely recommended in feline donors. Each cat donor should have a minimally acceptable PCV of 30%, although 35–40% is preferred.

BLOOD TYPING

Prior to administering blood products, knowledge of the donor and recipient's blood types, and a cross-match procedure, should be performed, as time allows. As a minimum, blood typing should be performed prior to administration. Rapid blood typing cards are available for use in dogs and cats (Rapid-Vet™ Feline and Canine blood typing cards, DMS Laboratories, Flemington, NJ, **80, 81**). The card test appears to be accurate for identifying DEA 1.1-positive and DEA 1.1-negative dogs, although some cross-reactivity with DEA 1.2 can occur, causing equivocal results.[7,8] In cats, the card test appears to be sensitive for identification of type A or type B, but is less

Table 19
Recommended screening tests for feline blood donors[4]

Disease	Infective organism	Test
FeLV	Feline leukemia virus	ELISA
FIV	Feline immunodeficiency virus	ELISA
Hemoplasmosis	*Mycoplasma haemofelis*	PCR, blood smears
	Mycoplasma haemominutum	PCR, blood smears
Bartonellosis	*Bartonella henselae*	IFA, PCR, culture
	Bartonella clarridgeae	IFA, PCR, culture
	Bartonella kholerae	IFA, PCR, culture

ELISA: enzyme-linked immunosorbent assay; IFA: immunofluorescent assay; PCR: polymerase chain reaction.

sensitive for type AB cats.[7,8] If equivocal results occur, the donor or recipient's blood should be sent to an outside laboratory for more definitive testing and typing.[7] Because the card test screens for agglutination, animals that are autoagglutinating cannot be typed using this method. A newer blood typing test is more specific for determining DEA 1.1-positive versus DEA 1.1-negative dogs, and type A from type B cats (DEA Vet Blood Type Kits, Vetscan, Abaxis, Union City, CA, USA) (**82**). An advantage of this method is that unlike blood typing cards that cannot be used in animals that are autoagglutinating, and that can also be subjective in nature, the newer well test is performed with the patient's serum, and is not affected by the presence of autoagglutination.

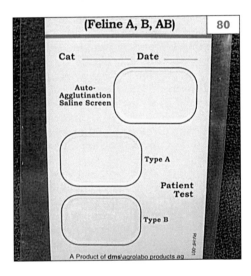

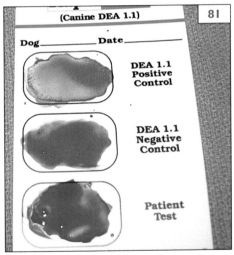

80 Rapid blood typing. The patient's whole blood is mixed with antibodies impregnated onto the card. Once read, the patient's blood type is known;

81 Rapid blood typing. The DEA 1.1-positive control shows agglutination, and below, a DEA 1.1-negative control does not. The dog's blood on the bottom of the card has no agglutination, and most closely resembles the DEA 1.1-negative control, so the dog is DEA 1.1 negative.

82 Blood typing kit which can be used if autoagglutination is present.

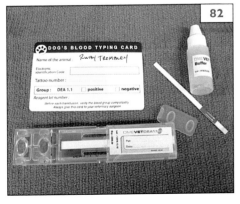

Canine blood groups

Dog erythrocytes contain various glycolipid and glycoprotein moieties on the cell surface that trigger an antigenic response. These protein and carbohydrate moieties are known as DEAs and allow the classification of blood types, or DEA subgroups (**83**). A total of 12 DEAs have been described, but the DEA subgroups 1.1, 1.2, 3, 4, 5, and 7 can be tested with antisera.[3] The most antigenic protein is DEA 1.1. Other antigenically important DEA subgroups include DEA 1.2, 4, and 7, but although these can cause some reactivity, there are not as important as DEA 1.1 in causing a transfusion reaction unless a dog has been sensitized from an earlier blood transfusion.[8] Ideally, dogs that are negative for DEA 1.1 and positive for only DEA 4 are known as 'universal donors'.[3] A benefit of having both DEA 1.1-positive and DEA 1.1-negative donors is that type-specific whole blood and type-specific packed red blood cells (pRBCs) can be administered to dogs, and increase the donor pool in the blood bank. Most recently, a report of a Dalmatian[9] and a type A feline renal transplant recipient[10,11] that required multiple cross-matches before a compatible donor was found, revealed the discovery of a new blood type in the dog (Dal) and cat (Mik). Although the blood types may be rare, the discoveries suggest a need to perform both a blood type and a cross-match before administration of any RBC product.[12] The general practitioner must determine the likelihood of a dog or cat having one of these very rare blood types and weigh the risks of transfusion with the perceived need for a cross-match or simply administering type-specific blood to a first-time recipient of a blood transfusion.

Feline blood groups

Cats have three naturally occurring blood types: A, B, and AB (**84**).[13,14] Unlike dogs, cats have naturally occurring antibodies directed against other feline blood types. In the majority of domestic cats within the USA and Great Britain, the predominant blood type is type A.[15] Type A cats have small quantities of naturally occurring antibodies directed against type B blood. Transfusion of type B blood into a type A cat will usually not cause a life-threatening reaction, but will greatly reduce the life-span of the transfused blood to only 2–3 days.[13–15]

Specialty breeds such as the British Shorthair, Devon Rex, and Ragdoll cats have a higher percentage of type B cats than the general domestic cat population. However, type B domestic shorthaired cats do occur. Type B domestic cats are much less common than type A cats except in areas of the Pacific Northwest USA, France, and Australia.[15] In the Pacific Northwest USA, the prevalence of type B cats has been reported to be up to 6%,[15,16] 15% in France,[15] and 73% in Australia.[16] Type B cats have large quantities of naturally occurring antibodies directed against type A blood. Infusion of type A blood into a type B cat can cause a life-threatening hemolytic transfusion reaction, including hypotension, bradycardia, apparent anxiety, depression, coagulopathy, and hemoglobinuria.[14–16] Because of the potential to cause death in any cat that is transfused with the incorrect blood type, ALL cats must have a blood type performed, and receive type-specific blood for a transfusion, without exception.

Type AB cats are rare, and have been documented in only 0.14% of cats in the USA and Canada.[17–19] Cats with blood type AB do not contain any naturally occurring antibodies directed against type A or type B blood. For this reason, the type AB cat is a 'universal feline recipient',[17–19] and theoretically can receive either type A or type B blood if in need of a RBC transfusion. However, hemolytic transfusion reactions have occurred when type B blood was infused into a type AB cat, so transfusion of AB cats with type A blood is recommended.[19] Finally, a Mik antigen has been documented in some cats. Cats that are Mik-negative are thought to produce alloantibodies against Mik-positive blood. Therefore, transfusion of Mik-positive blood to a Mik-negative cat can result in a transfusion reaction.[11]

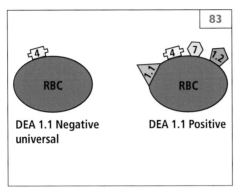

83 Diagram of canine blood types, showing various antigens on the surface of the red blood cell. DEA 1.1 negative is considered to be a 'universal donor'.

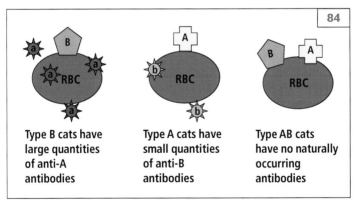

84 Diagram of feline blood types. Type A is most common, followed by type B, then type AB. An extremely rare Mik type has been documented. Type B cats have large quantities of naturally occurring autoantibodies against type A blood. Type A cats have small amounts of naturally occurring autoantibodies against type B blood. Type AB cats have no naturally occurring autoantibodies, and are the 'universal recipient' of the cat world.

CROSS-MATCH PROCEDURE

A cross-match procedure simulates *in vitro* the response of a recipient to donor plasma and RBC antigens. The cross-match procedure is performed to decrease the risk of transfusion reactions in patients that have been previously sensitized, that have naturally occurring alloantibodies, or in situations of neonatal isoerythrolysis. Other indications for cross-matching include decreasing the risk of sensitizing a patient if more than one transfusion is anticipated. After 5 days a dog or cat can produce antibodies to the antigens in the transfused blood. If more than 5 days has elapsed from the time of the first transfusion, a cross-match is required to determine whether the donor and recipient blood combinations are compatible.

Cross-matching can be divided into major and minor categories. The major cross-match mixes the donor's RBCs with recipient's plasma, thus testing whether the recipient contains antibodies against donor RBCs. A minor cross-match mixes donor plasma with recipient RBCs, testing for the unlikely occurrence that the donor serum contains antibodies directed against recipient RBCs. The cross-match procedures do not check for other sources of immediate hypersensitivity transfusion reactions, including white blood cell and platelets. There is a commercially available kit for cross-matching, but is not as sensitive or specific as the more labor-intensive in-house laboratory mixing of donor and recipient blood cells and plasma (**85**, *Table 20*).

Table 20
Cross-matching protocol

Supplies needed: 0.9% physiologic saline in wash bottle
   3 mL test tubes
   Pasteur pipettes
   Centrifuge
   Agglutination viewer lamp
1. Label test tubes as follows
     RC recipient control
     RR recipient RBCs
     RP recipient plasma
     DB donor whole blood*
     DC donor control*
     DR donor RBCs*
     DP donor plasma*
     Ma major cross-match*
     Mi minor cross-match*
* Indicates that this must be done for each donor being tested.
2. Obtain a cross-match segment from blood bank refrigerator for each donor to be cross-matched, or use an EDTA tube of donor's blood. MAKE SURE TUBES ARE LABELED PROPERLY.
3. Collect 2 mL of blood from recipient and place in an EDTA tube. Centrifuge for 5 minutes.

4. Extract blood from donor tubing. Centrifuge for 5 minutes. Use a separate pipette for each transfer, as cross-contamination can occur.
5. Pipette plasma off donor and recipient cells and place in tubes labeled DP and RP, respectively.
6. Place 125 μL donor and recipient cells in tubes labeled DR and RR, respectively.
7. Add 2.5 mL 0.9% NaCl solution from wash bottle to each RBC tube, using some force to cause cells to mix.
8. Centrifuge RBC suspension for 2 minutes.
9. Discard supernatant and resuspend RBCs with 0.9% NaCl from wash bottle.
10. Repeat steps 8 and 9 for a total of 3 washes.
11. Place 2 drops of donor RBC suspension and 2 drops of recipient plasma in tube labeled Ma (major cross-match).
12. Place 2 drops of donor plasma and 2 drops recipient RBC suspension in tube labeled Mi (minor cross-match).
13. Prepare control tubes by placing 2 drops donor plasma with 2 drops donor RBC suspension (This is the donor control); and place 2 drops recipient plasma with 2 drops recipient RBC suspension (This is the recipient control).
14. Incubate major and minor cross-matches and control tubes at room temperature for 15 minutes.
15. Centrifuge all tubes for 1 minute.
16. Read tubes using an agglutination viewer.
17. Check for agglutination and/or hemolysis (85)
18. Score agglutination with the following scoring scale:
    4+ one solid clump of cells
    3+ several large clumps of cells
    2+ medium-sized clumps of cells with a clear background
    1+ hemolysis, no clumping of cells
    NEG   negative for hemolysis; negative for clumping of red blood cells.

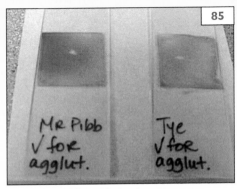

85 Checking for agglutination.

BLOOD COLLECTION

Canine donor

Any blood collection should be performed in a manner that is least stressful for the donor animal. A physical examination, PCV and total solids (PCV/TS) should be performed prior to any donation. Blood can be obtained from a jugular vein or femoral artery. However, due to the risk of lacerating the femoral artery, with subsequent hemorrhage or the development of compartmental syndrome, the jugular vein should be the primary site of blood collection in both dogs and cats. To collect blood, the fur is clipped over the jugular vein, taking care to avoid causing abrasions on the skin. Dogs should be placed in lateral recumbency; however, sternal recumbency or sitting on the floor are also acceptable methods. The area over the clipped jugular vein is scrubbed aseptically to avoid bacterial contamination of the donor and blood product. Next, the blood is collected into a closed system. Closed collection systems reduce the potential for contamination of the blood product, and facilitate the processing of blood components. Closed collection systems can be purchased from commercial blood banks such as Animal Blood Resources International (**86**). The blood collected is then mixed with an anticoagulant such as citrate–phosphate–dextrose–adenine (CPDA; 63 mL per 400–450 mL blood collected).[3] Whole blood mixed with anticoagulant alone, such as CPDA, remains viable for transfusion for 32 days. If the blood or pRBC are further mixed with a preservative such as Optisol, which contains mannitol, adenine, sodium chloride, and dextrose, the cells will remain viable for up to 42 days. After these recommended time frames, the product should be discarded.

To obtain a unit of blood from a donor dog, a 16 gauge needle is gently inserted into the jugular vein (**87**). The collection system is placed on a scale on the floor, and zeroed (**88**). The hemostat on the collection tubing can then be removed, and the blood is collected by gravity flow, or the blood collection bag is placed in a suction chamber to allow more rapid withdrawal of blood from the donor. Canine units should be approximately 450 mL, which translates to 450 g on the tared scale, since 1 mL weighs approximately 1 g. Although a volume of 450 mL can be obtained every 21 days, if necessary, from a healthy canine donor, less frequent donating of every 2–3 months is preferred. If a large dog (>132 lb [60 kg]) has donated two units (900 mL) at a time, a minimum of 6 weeks should elapse before the next donation. The estimated circulating blood volume in a dog is 90 mL/kg. Dogs can lose up to 20% of their circulating blood volume before clinical signs of hypovolemia occur. However, it is prudent to take only 500–1000 mL of blood, depending on the size of the donor. Once the blood sample has been collected, a bandage should be placed over the venipuncture site for a minimum of 1 hour, until a clot has formed. Unless the donor is showing signs of hypovolemia, such as tachycardia, pale mucous membranes, or poor pulse quality, intravenous or subcutaneous fluids are not necessary.

Feline donor

Feline blood collection often requires the use of sedation, unless a permanent vascular access port (VAP) port has been surgically implanted. All donor cats should have a physical examination and PCV/TS performed prior to sedation and subsequent blood donation. In most cases, donor cats are heavily sedated or anesthetized (ketamine/diazepam, propofol, or gas anesthesia) prior to collection of the blood for transfusion. Following sedation or anesthesia, depending on the temperament of the cat and hospital policy, the fur over the jugular vein is clipped and the area aseptically scrubbed. A 19 gauge butterfly catheter is inserted into the jugular vein and aspirated with gentle pressure into a 60 mL syringe into which 7 mL of CPDA or acid–citrate–dextrose (ACD) anticoagulant has been placed (**89**). In most cases, a total volume of 53 mL of blood is obtained. The blood can be immediately transfused, or placed into a small sterile collection bag for storage for up to 32 days. No more than 11–15 mL/kg should be obtained at any given time from a feline donor. Following donation, if a cat shows signs of hypovolemia, such as poor pulse quality, tachycardia or pale mucous membranes, intravenous fluids can be administered.

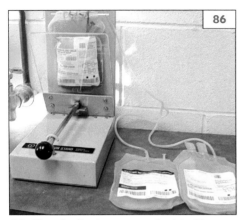

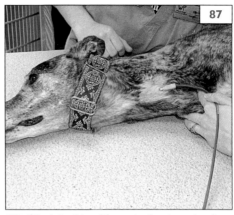

86 Closed collection system of original bag into which blood is obtained, which then can be separated out into two satellite bags, one for packed red blood cells, and one for plasma.

87 Obtaining blood from the jugular vein of a greyhound blood donor.

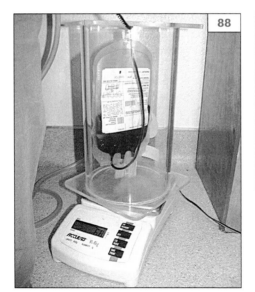

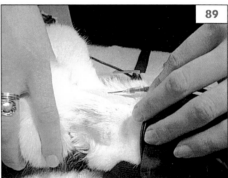

89 Cat placed in dorsal recumbency, with needle inserted into the external jugular vein for blood donation.

88 Photo of a vacuum chamber on a tared scale. Suction on the vacuum chamber helps hasten the procurement of a blood donation.

BLOOD COMPONENTS

Processing and storage

Blood component therapy has become more commonplace in both human and veterinary medicine. Component therapy involves the separation of whole blood into its cellular and plasma components, then administering specific components to a recipient based on each patient's individual needs. Preparation of fresh frozen plasma (FFP), frozen plasma (FP), cryoprecipitate, and cryo-poor plasma requires the use of a refrigerated centrifuge. Floor and table-top refrigerated centrifuge models are currently available for purchase. In many cases, purchase of a refrigerated centrifuge is impractical due to expense and space required for its storage. A veterinary community can potentially pool resources for the cost of the equipment and house the unit at a centrally located facility, such as a local emergency hospital. Alternatively, human hospitals or blood banks may provide separation services for a nominal fee.

Once obtained, blood should be collected into a plastic bag system designed specifically for blood collection. The blood should be stripped from the collection tubing, and the line can then be sealed using a thermal seal or aluminum clips (**90**, *Tables 21, 22*). The bag should be clearly labeled with the donor's name, blood type, the date of collection, the donor's PCV at the time of collection, and expiration date. If the blood is not going to be used immediately or prepared for platelet-rich plasma, it should be refrigerated until used or until it has expired. The unit can also be separated into fresh plasma and pRBC components by centrifugation in a refrigerated centrifuge (4000–5000 g for 15 minutes). Following centrifugation, a plasma extractor will facilitate flow of plasma into designated satellite bags for further storage of the FFP (**91, 92**).

FFP, cryoprecipitate, and cryo-poor plasma should be frozen within 8 hours of collection to ensure preservation of labile clotting factors, including factors V, VIII, and von Willebrand factor (VWf). FFP has a shelf-life of 1 year after the date of collection. Partial thawing and differential centrifugation of FFP allows preparation of cryoprecipitate and cryo-poor plasma. After 1 year, or if a unit of plasma has

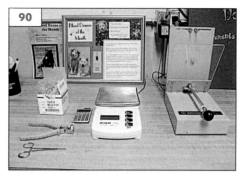

90 Scale, hemostat forceps, roller clamp used to strip the line of collection bags, and separation device used to separate whole blood into plasma and packed red blood cells.

Table 21
Supplies needed for canine blood collection and storage

Blood donor collection bag
Sealing clips
Pliers or tube stripper (optional)
Guarded hemostat
Plasma press
Refrigerated centrifuge
Storage freezer
Storage refrigerator

Table 22
Supplies needed for feline blood collection and storage

60 mL syringe
3-way stop-cock
7 mL CPDA anticoagulant solution
20 gauge needle
Storage refrigerator

been prepared 8 hours after collection, FP results. FP contains all of the vitamin K-dependent coagulation factors (II, VII, IX, X), immunoglobulins, and albumin, but is relatively devoid of the labile clotting factors. FP has a shelf-life of 5 years after the original date of collection, or 4 years after expiration of a unit of FFP. Packed RBCs should be stored at 1–6ºC immediately after collection and processing. FP and pRBCs can also be prepared in the absence of a refrigerated centrifuge by storing the unit of whole blood upright in a 1–6ºC refrigerator for 12–24 hours, until the RBCs have separated out. The plasma can be drawn off into a second storage bag and frozen as FP. Due to the delay in processing, the resultant plasma does not contain the labile clotting factors. FFP, FP, cryoprecipitate, and cryo-poor plasma should be stored at −20ºC until use. The products should be thawed in tepid water until no crystals are observed. No plasma product should be heated to more than 37ºC, as protein denaturation can occur.

Platelets can remain viable for up to 8 hours at room temperature in CPDA-treated whole blood. An infusion of 10 mL/kg fresh whole blood will typically raise the recipient's platelet count approximately 10,000 platelets/μL. Platelet-rich plasma and platelet concentrate can be purchased from commercial blood banks, and usually delivers 5000–40,000 platelets to the recipient if 1 platelet unit per 10 kg is administered. Platelet-rich plasma must be stored according to specific recommendations from the blood bank. Unfortunately, due to the lag time in purchase and transport of the platelet product, it may be cost-prohibitive to infuse adequate number of platelets to retard bleeding in a severely thrombocytopenic animal.

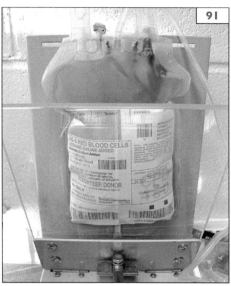

91 Whole blood after centrifugation that has been placed in an extractor device. Slow pressure on the bag of centrifuged whole blood helps separate whole blood into plasma and packed red blood cells.

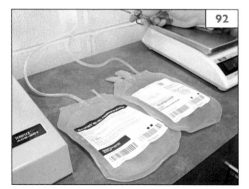

92 Forceps on the line that leads to the satellite bag for packed red blood cells allows separation of the plasma (on right) into one bag. After the plasma is collected into its satellite bag, that bag is tied off from the system, and the remaining red blood cells are decanted into the other satellite bag designated for them, which contains AC-D Optisol to prevent the cells from coagulating, and also to provide nourishment and stabilization for the red blood cells during storage.

Component therapy

(*Table 23*, **93**)

WHOLE BLOOD

Whole blood is collected from the donor animal, mixed with an anticoagulant, and then stored in a refrigerator until use. After collection, whole blood contains red and white blood cells, platelets, clotting factors, and other serum proteins, including immunoglobulin and albumin.[3] In dogs, approximately 450–500 mL of blood is obtained directly from the donor and collected into a sterile plastic satellite bag

Table 23
Blood component therapy

Blood product	Components	Uses	Dose
Whole blood	Red blood cells Clotting factors Albumin Globulins Platelets (small amount)	Anemia Acute blood loss	10–22 mL/kg
pRBCs	Red blood cells Plasma (small amount)	Anemia	6–10 mL/kg
Fresh frozen plasma	Clotting factors Albumin Globulin Antithrombin $\bar{\text{-}}$2 macroglobulin	Vitamin K antagonist rodenticide Hemophilias von Willebrand's disease	10–20 mL/kg
Cryoprecipitate	von Willebrand factor	von Willebrand's disease Hemophilia Vitamin K antagonist rodenticide	1 unit/10 kg body weight
Cryo-poor plasma	Coagulation factors II, VII, IX, X	Vitamin K antagonist rodenticide intoxication	1 unit/10 kg body weight
Platelet-rich plasma	Platelet suspension	Thrombocytopenia	Platelets from 1 unit of whole blood per 10 kg body weight
Frozen platelet concentrate	Platelets	Thrombocytopenia	1 unit/10 kg body weight will raise platelet count by 20,000

that contains 63 mL of an anticoagulant with nutrients such as CPDA.[3] This blood can be labeled and stored in a refrigerator until use or until it becomes expired. Typically, when stored at 6°C, whole blood remains viable for 4 weeks (28 days).[20] If no nutrients such as sodium citrate are present with the anticoagulant, the blood must be used immediately for infusion into the recipient (*Table 24*).

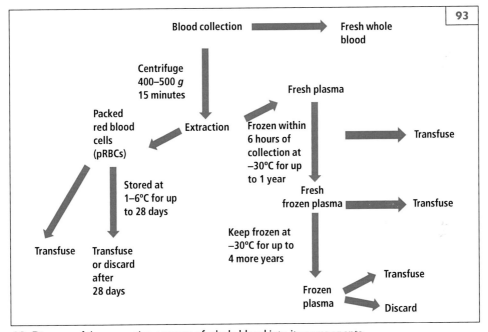

93 Diagram of the separation process of whole blood into its components.

Table 24
Anticoagulants and anticoagulant/preservatives for use in canine and feline blood collection and storage[2]

Anticoagulant	Ratio to blood	Storage
Heparin	625 units/50 mL	Use immediately
3.8% NaCitrate	1 mL/9 mL blood	Use immediately
Anticoagulant / preservative	*Ratio to blood*	*Storage*
ACD 'B' additive solutions	1 mL/7–9 mL blood	21 days canine
		30 days feline
ACD 'B' Additive solutions	100 mL/250 mL pRBCs	37–42 days canine

THE 'TRANSFUSION TRIGGER'

It is a common misconception that administration of whole blood or pRBCs should occur when patient PCV decreases to a certain number. In fact, no absolute 'transfusion trigger' number actually exists.[21] A transfusion should be administered whenever a patient demonstrates clinical signs of anemia, including lethargy, anorexia, weakness, tachycardia, and/or tachypnea. Indications for fresh whole blood transfusion include disorders of hemostasis and coagulopathies, including DIC, von Willebrand's disease, and hemophilia. Fresh whole blood and platelet-rich plasma can also be administered in cases of severe thrombocytopenia and thrombocytopathia. Stored whole blood and pRBCs can be administered to patients with anemia. In a retrospective study of over 600 blood transfusions in 300 canine recipients, reasons for transfusion included hemorrhage, hemolysis, and ineffective erythropoiesis.[21] If PCV drops to below 10% or if rapid hemorrhage causes the PCV to drop below 20% in the dog or less than 12–15% in the cat, a transfusion is advocated. FFP or cryoprecipitate administration should be considered in cases of coagulopathy, including von Willebrand's disease, rodenticide intoxication with depletion of activated vitamin K-dependent coagulation factors, hemophilia, or in cases of severe hypoproteinemia with albumin concentrations less than 2.0 g/dL (20 g/L). FP will suffice in cases of severe hypoproteinemia, warfarin-like compound intoxication, and factor IX deficiency (hemophilia B).

PACKED RED BLOOD CELLS

Packed red blood cells (pRBCs) are obtained when a unit of whole blood is centrifuged and separated from the plasma component. pRBCs contain a very small amount of plasma, anticoagulant, RBCs, platelets, and white blood cells. The platelets and white blood cells are insignificant in quantity and have a very short life-span once taken from the donor, so are essentially negligible. The PCV of pRBCs ranges from 60% to 80%, depending on the amount of plasma extracted from the unit during separation.[21] pRBCs should be administered in euvolemic animals with anemia that do not require clotting factors, albumin, or a significant amount of platelets. The recommended dose of pRBCs is 6–10 mL/kg.[4] Although some authors recommend resuspending units of pRBCs with 0.9% saline (10 mL saline to 40 mL pRBC product), this author has infused pRBCs without resuspension without complication.

FRESH FROZEN PLASMA (FFP)

FFP is the fluid component of whole blood that contains clotting factors, antithrombin, albumin, globulin, and α-2 macroglobulin after the cellular components have been centrifuged and separated. Plasma that has been frozen within 6 hours of collection is known as FFP, and retains labile clotting factors for 1 year if stored at −30ºC. FFP bags should be crimped with an elastic band prior to freezing, then frozen in a cardboard box to prevent accidental cracking of the plastic bag. Once the plasma is frozen, the elastic band should be removed. This will leave a 'cinched' area around the middle of the plasma (**94**). In the case of an inadvertent power cut, the crimp will expand if the plasma has thawed then refrozen before the power cut is discovered. This is an insurance policy to maintain the integrity and quality of the plasma product for the patient. Plasma that is frozen more than 6 hours after collection, or FFP that has been stored at −30ºC for more than 1 year is known as FP.[21] FP is deficient in some of the labile clotting factors, but is still viable for an additional 4 years at −30ºC. Before infusion, FFP and FP should be thawed to body temperature in a warm water (37ºC) bath. In some cases, microfractures or cracks in the plasma's plastic bag are not visible until the bag is thawed. The plasma should be placed in a separate plastic bag during the thawing process. If a crack and hence potential bacterial contamination of the product is present, the plasma will thaw and leak into the outer plastic bag, and become visible to the veterinary staff.

CRYOPRECIPITATE

Cryoprecipitate is the product obtained from partially thawing FFP at 0–6ºC, then centrifuging. At this temperature, a precipitate of VWf, factors XIII, VIII, and fibrinogen distributes on the bottom of the collection bag. This product is collected and can be refrozen for later use, or can be used immediately upon further thawing. The supernatant can also be collected and refrozen as cryo-poor plasma. Because cryoprecipitate contains large quantities of clotting factors in a relatively small fluid volume, the solution is considered the gold standard for the treatment of hemophilia A and von Willebrand's disease in very small animals. In larger dogs, the same factors can be administered as FFP, when intravascular volume overload is not a concern. A recommended dose of cryoprecipitate is 1 unit per 10 kg body weight,[4] or 12–20 mL/kg every 12 hours.[21]

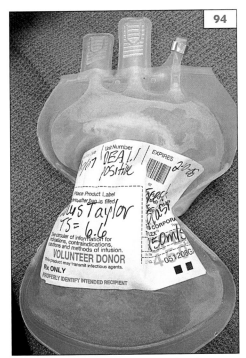

94 Fresh frozen plasma. An elastic band was secured around the bag before freezing, then removed after the freezing was complete. If there is inadvertent thawing of the bag, for example during a power outage, the 'crimp' in the bag will be gone, allowing the caregiver to know that the bag was thawed, then refrozen.

PLATELET-RICH PLASMA

Platelet-rich plasma is a product that is obtained by centrifuging fresh whole blood at a slower rate than when separating out RBCs from the plasma components.[3] The platelets are resuspended in a small amount of plasma, then stored in plastic bags at 20–24ºC under constant rocking.[3] The platelets administered are extremely labile, and are rapidly destroyed once infused into the recipient. A recommended dose of 1 unit of platelet-rich plasma should be administered per 10 kg body weight.[3] In many cases, numerous units are required to make a transient significant difference in platelet numbers in dogs that are actively bleeding from immune-mediated thrombocytopenia, for example. For this reason, the use of platelet-rich plasma is not common, and is sometimes cost-prohibitive.

CRYO-POOR PLASMA

Cryo-poor plasma is the supernatant that is collected and refrozen after partial thawing of FFP at 0–6ºC, centrifuged, and separated from VWf, factor XIII, factor VIII, and fibrinogen. The resultant solution is relatively devoid of these factors, but still contains the vitamin K-dependent coagulation factors II, VII, IX, and X.[4] Thus, cryo-poor plasma is ideal for the treatment of vitamin K antagonist rodenticide intoxication. The recommended dose of cryo-poor plasma is 10 mL/kg.[3] This can be repeated until coagulation abnormalities normalize.

FROZEN PLATELET CONCENTRATE

Frozen platelet concentrate is a solution that is obtained when platelets are collected from a donor via platelet pheresis, then mixed with dimethylsulfoxide preservative solution. One bag of frozen platelet concentrate contains approximately 1×10^{11} platelets. A recommended dose is 1 unit of frozen platelet concentrate per 10 kg body weight to increase the recipient's platelet count by 10–20,000 platelets/µL.[3]

HEMOGLOBIN-BASED OXYGEN CARRIERS

In the past decade, hemoglobin-based oxygen carriers (HBOCs) became more widely used in veterinary medicine. However, they are no longer available. Oxyglobin was a stroma-free, purified bovine hemoglobin product originally approved for use in dogs in 1998. The use of Oxyglobin became popular among private practitioners for a wide variety of reasons, including lack of need to keep donor blood readily available, long shelf-life, and decreased risk of transfusion reactions, antigenic stimulation, and disease transmission. Further advantages of Oxyglobin administration included its potent colloid effect, improved oxygen delivery, and improved blood rheology. Recommended doses for dogs ranged from 10 to 30 mL/kg. An average dose of 15 mL/kg had an effect for approximately 24–48 hours. Indications for HBOC administration included hookworm-related anemia, flea-anemia, immune-mediated hemolytic anemia, and massive hemorrhage. Contraindications for their use included congestive heart failure, anuric renal failure, and intravascular volume overload, as pulmonary edema could ensue, thus increasing patient morbidity and mortality. One study published results of HBOC use in cats in a large referral teaching hospital. An average dose of 14.6 mL/kg was administered to 72 cats, with an incidence of 44 adverse reactions. The most severe reactions included the development of pulmonary edema and pleural effusion. Following administration of an HBOC, plasma and urine may appear port-wine colored for several days (**95**). This can affect any colorimetric test used for serum biochemistry analysis.

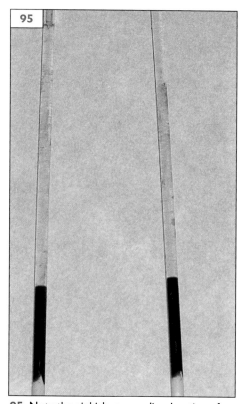

95 Note the pinkish orange discoloration of the plasma in these hematocrit tubes. This patient had received a hemoglobin-based oxygen carrier.

TRANSFUSION THERAPY

Indications

There are many indications for administering transfusions of whole blood and component blood products. Conditions that commonly require administration of whole blood or blood component therapy include anemia secondary to loss of whole blood (e.g. hemorrhage), immune-mediated hemolytic anemia, bone marrow aplasia or chronic severe renal failure with lack of erythropoiesis, coagulation disorders, and hypoproteinemia.[22]

A step-wise approach should be taken for every patient that may require a transfusion. If a patient is at risk for blood loss, or is anemic, a transfusion should be considered. A decision should be made on the type of transfusion therapy appropriate for each particular patient. Once a decision is made about which components need to be administered, the clinician should calculate a volume to be delivered. Caution should be exercised when administering larger volumes to small patients or those with cardiac insufficiency, as volume overload with subsequent pulmonary edema can potentially occur. If RBC products are to be administered, a minimum of a blood typing should be performed before giving type-specific blood. The gold standard is to perform a cross-match for each unit administered, to reduce the risk of a transfusion reaction or sensitizing the patient to foreign RBC antigens. In some cases of severe hemorrhage when there is not enough time to perform even a blood typing, universal blood (DEA 1.1, 1.2, and 7 negative) can be administered.

Administration of blood products

Blood products should slowly be warmed to 37ºC before administering to the patient. Blood warmer units are available for use in veterinary medicine to facilitate rapid transfusion without reducing patient body temperature. RBC and plasma products should be administered in a blood administration set containing a 170–270 μm in-line filter.[21] Smaller in-line filters (18 μm, Hemo-Nate blood filter, Utah Medical Products, Midvale,

UT) can also be used, in cases where extremely small volumes are to be administered. Blood products should be administered over a period of 4 hours, whenever possible, according to guidelines set by the American Association of Blood Banks. In cases where there is acute, life-threatening hemorrhage and hypovolemia, blood products can also be administered as a rapid bolus. A recommended dose of whole blood in dogs is 10–22 mL/kg.[3] As a general rule, administration of 1 mL fresh or stored whole blood per pound (2 mL/kg) will raise the recipient's PCV by 1 percentage point, provided that no ongoing loss or hemorrhage is present (the 'Rule of Ones').

To calculate the amount of whole blood transfusion to administer, the following equations are used:

$$\text{Dog: Transfusion (mL)} = \frac{\text{Weight (lb)} \times 40 \times (\text{desired PCV} - \text{patient PCV})/\text{donor PCV}}{[\text{Weight (kg)} \times 18.1]}$$

$$\text{Cat: Transfusion (mL)} = \frac{\text{Weight (lb)} \times 30 \times (\text{desired PCV} - \text{patient PCV})/\text{donor PCV}}{[\text{Weight (kg)} \times 13.6]}$$

Administration of half that volume of pRBCs will have a similar effect on recipient PCV, unless ongoing loss or hemorrhage is present. FFP, FP, and cryoprecipitate should be administered at a volume of 10 mL/kg until bleeding is controlled or ongoing albumin loss ceases. The goal of transfusion therapy should be to raise the PCV to 25–30% in dogs, and 15–20% in cats, or to raise the albumin to a minimum of 2.0 g/dL (20 g/L), or until bleeding stops as in the case of coagulopathies. Monitoring of the patient to ensure that bleeding has stopped, coagulation profiles (ACT, APTT, and prothrombin time [PT]) have normalized, hypovolemia has stabilized, and/or total protein is normalizing is necessary before discontinuing ongoing transfusion therapy.

Fresh and stored whole blood and pRBCs should appear red in color, similar to a venous blood sample. If the blood product has brown, purple, or green discoloration, bacterial contamination should be suspected, and the unit should not be infused into the recipient.[3] Blood products can be infused either intravenously or via intraosseous catheterization. Large volumes of blood products should be administered through a 170 μm filter in a blood administration set. Smaller, 18 μm in-line filters can be used for small volumes of plasma and RBCs. Ideally, the blood or plasma product should be administered very slowly during the first half hour of infusion (0.25 mL/kg).[3] If no transfusion reaction is observed, the rate can then be increased to allow the desired calculated volume to be infused over the next 4 hours. Plasma can be administered at a slightly higher rate of 4–6 mL/minute if necessary to reverse a coagulopathy.

Monitoring during transfusion (96)

Several studies have documented the incidence of transfusion reactions in dogs and cats.[22] Overall, the incidence of transfusion reactions is 2.5% in dogs, and 2% in cats. With careful donor selection, knowledge of the recipient and donor blood types, and utilization of cross-match procedures for recipients that have received prior transfusions, the incidence of transfusion reactions can be dramatically reduced.[22] Transfusion reactions can be immune-mediated and nonimmune-mediated in nature, and can happen immediately, or can be delayed after a transfusion. Acute reactions usually occur within minutes to hours of the onset of transfusion, but may occur up to 48 hours after the transfusion has been completed or discontinued. Acute immunologic reactions include hemolysis, vomiting, fever, facial swelling, ptyalism, urticaria, and neonatal isoerythrolysis.[2,23] Signs of a delayed immunologic reaction include hemolysis, purpura, and immunosuppression.

Acute nonimmunologic reactions include donor cell hemolysis prior to onset of transfusion, circulatory volume overload, bacterial contamination, citrate toxicity with clinical signs of hypocalcemia, coagulopathies, hyperammonemia, hypothermia, air embolism, acidosis, and pulmonary microembolism. Delayed nonimmunologic reactions include the transmission and development of infectious diseases, and hemosiderosis. Clinical signs of a transfusion reaction typically depend on the amount of blood transfused, the type and amount of antibody involved in the reaction, and whether the recipient has had previous sensitization. There has been one report of a massive transfusion reaction to DEA 1.1 in a dog that had previous transfusions from a compatible donor.[23]

Monitoring the patient carefully during the transfusion period is essential in recognizing early signs of a transfusion reaction, including those that may become life-threatening. A general guideline for patient monitoring is to start the transfusion slowly during the first 15 minutes. Temperature, pulse, and respiration should be monitored every 15 minutes for the first hour, 1 hour after the end of the transfusion, and at a minimum of every 12 hours thereafter. The most common documented clinical signs of a transfusion reaction include pyrexia, urticaria, salivation/ptyalism, nausea, chills, and vomiting.[24] Other clinical signs may include tachycardia, tremors, collapse, dyspnea, weakness, hypotension, collapse, or seizures. Severe intravascular hemolytic reactions may occur within minutes of the start of the transfusion, causing hemoglobinemia, hemoglobinuria, DIC, and clinical signs of shock. Extravascular hemolytic reactions typically occur later, and will result in hyperbilirubinemia and bilirubinuria. In many cases, nausea and vomiting associated with administration of RBC products is caused by ammonia accumulation in the product, and is not a true anaphylactic reaction (*Table 25*).[24]

BLOOD TRANSFUSION WORKSHEET		
Patient Information		
Date:	Recipient:	Prior Pregnancy: Y/N
DVM:	Recipient PCV/TS:	Recipient Blood Type
Weight:	Prior Transfusion: Y/N	Diagnosis Reason for Transfusion

Blood Product Information

Cross-Match to Donor: Y/N	Donor Name:
Type of Blood Product	Donor Blood Type:
pRBCs / Fresh Whole Blood	Unit size (m/s):
Fresh Frozen Plasma	Unit PCV/TS:
Stored Whole Blood	Expiration Date of Unit:
Frozen Plasma	

Please note any urticaria, facial swelling, vomiting or pruritus at any time and notify DVM

Start Time:	Baseline	15 min	30 min	45 min	1 hr	2 hr	3 hr	4 hr
Administration Rate								
Temperature								
HR/RR								
mm color/CRT								

96 Example of a worksheet used for documentation of parameters and information during a blood transfusion.

Table 25
Clinical signs of transfusion reaction

Angioneurotic edema
Collapse
Diarrhea
Discolored (pink) plasma
Vomiting
Hemoglobinuria
Hemolysis
Hypotension
Ptyalism
Urticaria

Pre-treatment of patients to help reduce the risk of a transfusion reaction remains controversial, as in most cases pre-treatment with glucocorticoids and antihistamines is ineffective at preventing intravascular hemolysis and other reactions, should they occur. The most important component of preventing a transfusion reaction is to screen each recipient and carefully process the donor component therapy before the administration of any blood products.

Treatment of a transfusion reaction depends on its severity. In all cases, the transfusion should be immediately stopped when clinical signs of a reaction occurs. In most cases, discontinuing the transfusion and administering drugs such as diphenhydramine and famotidine to stop the hypersensitivity reaction will be sufficient (*Table 26*). Once the above medications have taken effect, the transfusion can be restarted slowly and the patient monitored carefully for further signs of reaction. In more severe cases in which a patient's cardiovascular or respiratory system become compromised, and hypotension, tachycardia, or tachypnea occur, the transfusion should be immediately discontinued, and diphenhydramine, dexamethasone-sodium phosphate, and epinephrine should be administered. The patient should have a urinary catheter and central venous catheter placed, for measurement of urine output and CVP. Aggressive fluid therapy may be necessary to avoid renal insufficiency or renal damage associated with severe intravascular hemolysis. Overhydration with subsequent pulmonary edema can generally be managed with supplemental oxygen administration and intravenous or intramuscular furosemide (2–4 mg/kg). Plasma products with or without heparin can be administered for DIC.

Monitoring after transfusion

Following infusion of blood products, it is important to evaluate the patient's clinical response to therapy. Guidelines for monitoring depend on the clinical condition for which the transfusion was required. A baseline patient PCV should be performed prior to the start of any transfusion. Following administration of pRBCs or whole blood, a PCV should be performed after the transfusion is complete, and every 12 hours thereafter. A general guideline is that the PCV should rise by 1 percentage point for each 1 mL/lb (2.2mL/kg) of whole blood administered. If the PCV is markedly lower than that calculated volume, ongoing loss in the form of hemorrhage or lysis should be considered. Coagulation parameters such as an ACT and platelet count should be monitored at least daily in patients requiring transfusion therapy.

Table 26
Treatment of transfusion reactions

Drug	Dose	Route
Diphenhydramine	1–2 mg/kg	IM
Dexamethasone-SP	0.5–1.0 mg/kg	IM or IV
Epinephrine	0.01 mg/kg	IV

When plasma products (FFP, FP, cryoprecipitate, cryo-poor plasma) have been administered for coagulation abnormalities, coagulation testing in the form of PT, APTT, and ACT should be performed after the transfusion finishes. Blood product administration can also be associated with dilutional coagulopathies and hypocalcemia. An ionized calcium should be performed whenever large volumes of blood products have been administered to a small animal patient, and the patient monitored closely for signs of hypocalcemia (facial twitching, seizures, refractory hypotension, prolonged QT interval on electrocardiogram).

When done correctly, administration of blood products can make the difference between life and death in a critically ill animal. In some animals, however, blood product administration can be associated with potentially life-threatening complications if care and forethought are not exercised prior to transfusion. Infusion of type A blood into a type B cat can result in rapid hemolysis and death.[10] In dogs, previous sensitization to RBCs from prior transfusion can result in hemolysis, pigmenturia, and hypotension if a blood type and cross-match are not performed.[2] Other transfusion reactions that have been described include ionized hypocalcemia, fever, vomiting, urticaria, angioneurotic edema, and hypotension.[2] Ionized hypocalcemia can make the vasculature less sensitive to circulating catecholamines, and potentiate vasodilation, cardiac dysfunction, hypothermia, and hypotension. If an animal develops refractory hypotension and hypothermia following the administration of blood products, citrate toxicity and ionized hypocalcemia must be considered. Treatment of hypocalcemia consists of replenishing calcium with the administration of calcium gluconate (1 mL/kg 10% slowly).[2] Dogs that have received massive transfusions, defined as a volume of blood products greater than the animal's blood volume (>90 mL/kg), have been shown to develop ionized hypocalcemia, thrombocytopenia, and coagulopathy.[20]

To help prevent a transfusion reaction, the patient's blood type should be obtained before administration of any blood product to a dog or cat. Ideally, a cross-match procedure should also be obtained to prevent adverse complications.[3] Nausea, ptyalism and vomiting can also be caused by the accumulation of nitrogenous waste products such as urea in stored blood.[25] Severe reactions that result in collapse and hypotension should be treated with rapid discontinuation of the blood product and prompt administration of epinephrine (0.01 mg/kg IV). There has been one report of the rare complication of iron toxicity, or hemochromatosis, reported in a Miniature Schnauzer with pure RBC aplasia that had received multiple RBC transfusions over several years.[26] There have been other reports of transmission of infectious diseases such as leishmaniasis to dogs from infected blood donors.[5,6]

Diagnosis and treatment of electrolyte abnormalities

- **Disorders of sodium**

- **Disorders of chloride**

- **Disorders of potassium**

- **Disorders of calcium**

- **Disorders of phosphorus**

- **Disorders of magnesium**

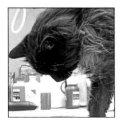
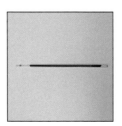
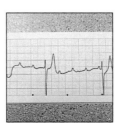

DISORDERS OF SODIUM

Sodium is a major extracellular cation that acts as an effective osmole, i.e. it does not cross cell membranes readily, and can exert osmotic effects across a gradient. Water will follow by osmosis across a cellular membrane, depending on the concentration of sodium on either side of the membrane. Water will move from an area of lower sodium (higher water) concentration to higher sodium sodium concentration. In patients with a variety of disease states, hypernatremia and hyponatremia are commonly observed.

Hyponatremia

Hyponatremia, by definition, is a serum concentration of sodium below normal reference ranges (*Table 27*), namely, less than 140 mEq/L. Causes of hyponatremia are listed in *Table 28*. Hyponatremia can be caused by excessive retention of water in excess of sodium. This is observed in animals with congestive heart failure, with activation of the renin–angiotensin–aldosterone axis. As water is retained, serum sodium becomes diluted. Another cause of hyponatremia is renal wasting of sodium, usually due to a lack of influence of aldosterone. In animals with hypoadrenocorticism, who lack aldosterone, sodium and water are not reabsorbed by the renal collecting tubules, and the animal becomes hyponatremic. With diabetes mellitus, glucose acts as an effective osmole and will cause water to move from the interstitial to the intravascular space and dilute the sodium present. In general, for every 100 mg/dL (5.55 mmol/L) increase in blood glucose above normal, serum sodium decreases by 1.6 mEq/L. The effect can be severe in hyperglycemic, hyperosmolar animals with diabetes mellitus. Animals also will become hyponatremic due to vomiting and diarrhea, third-spacing of fluids in pleural or peritoneal effusion, severe burn injuries, hepatic failure, nephritic syndrome, and psychogenic polydipsia. A syndrome of inappropriate ADH secretion (SIADH), which causes the release of arginine vasopressin (ADH) in the face of

Table 27
Normal electrolyte reference values

Electrolyte	Canine normal	Feline normal
Sodium (mEq/L)(mmol/L)	140.3–153.9	145.8–158.7
Chloride (mEq/L)(mmol/L)	102.1–117.4	107.5–129.6
Potassium (mEq/L)(mmol/L)	3.8–5.6	3.8–5.3
Total calcium (mg/dL)	8.7–11.8	7.9–10.9
(mmol/L)	2.2–3.0	2.0–2.7
Magnesium (mg/dL)	1.7–2.7	1.9–2.8
(mmol/L)	0.7–1.1	0.8–1.2
Phosphorus (mg/dL)	2.9–6.2	4.0–7.3
(mmol/L)	1.0–2.0	1.3–2.4

normal to low plasma osmolality results in retention of water and dilution of sodium. This syndrome is rare, but has been described in animals.

Clinical signs of hyponatremia often are lacking unless hyponatremia is severe (<120 mEq/L), and has developed very acutely in less than 24–48 hours. Severe and rapid decreases in serum sodium will cause the

Table 28
Causes of hyponatremia
Congestive heart failure
Renal failure/urinary loss
Third-spacing of fluid
Pleural effusion
Neoplasia
Lung lobe torsion
Chylothorax
Abdominal effusion
Chlyoabdomen
Neoplasia
Peritonitis
Pancreatitis
Uroabdomen
Burn injury
Hypoadrenocorticism
Pseudohypoadrenocorticism
Whipworm (*Trichuris* spp.) infestation
Pregnancy (Greyhounds)
Diuretic administration
SIADH
Hypothalamic tumor
Dirofilariasis
Carcinoma
Psychogenic polydipsia
Diabetes mellitus
Gastrointestinal loss
Vomiting
Diarrhea

intracellular space to become hyperosmolar with respect to the extracellular space. Fluid (water) moves from areas of lower to higher sodium concentrations in an attempt to make conditions iso-osmotic. As such, water will move into cells and cause cellular edema. This becomes particularly important in neuronal tissue such as the brain, where influx of water results in cerebral edema. Clinical signs of cerebral edema include ataxia, depression, lethargy, head pressing, seizures, and coma.

Treatment of clinical hyponatremia largely is directed at treating the primary cause, when possible. For example, treatment of hyperosmolar nonketotic diabetes mellitus and reduction in serum glucose with the administration of exogenous insulin will eventually result in normalization of serum sodium concentration once the diabetes mellitus is regulated. Treatment of the primary cause of abdominal or thoracic effusions, such as chylothorax, peritonitis, or neoplasia, or loss of sodium with burn injury can result in serum sodium becoming normalized once the effusion is no longer accumulating and the burns heal. Treatment of hypoadrenocorticism or pseudohypoadrenocorticism with exogenous sources of aldosterone (fludrocortisone acetate, or desoxycorticosterone pivalate [DOCP], for example), or treatment of gastrointestinal (GI) parasitism (e.g. whipworm infestation) and correction of the associated diarrhea, will result in normalization of serum sodium. In severe hyponatremia, particularly in animals whose serum sodium is less than 120 mEq/L, serum sodium must be corrected very carefully, to avoid raising the sodium by more than 1 mEq/L per hour, in general, over the first 24–48 hours. If serum sodium rises too quickly, and the hyponatremia has been long-standing, the rapid rise of serum sodium will be sensed as the cell being hypo-osmolar to the extracellular fluid, and water will rush out of the cells into the extracellular space. In neuronal tissue, the cell shrinkage is known as central pontine myelinolysis. Clinical signs usually occur several days after therapy, and are manifested by head pressing, ataxia, vocalization, lethargy, depression, seizures, coma, or death.

Hypernatremia

Hypernatremia is defined as serum sodium greater than normal reference ranges (more than 155 mEq/L).[1,2] Causes of hypernatremia are listed in *Table 29*. There are several possible mechanisms of hypernatremia. The most common mechanism of hypernatremia in small animals is a loss of water in excess of salt, which is also known as free water loss. Water loss can occur in the GI tract, as diarrhea, or in the kidneys due to osmotic diuresis or a lack of action of ADH (central or nephrogenic diabetes insipidus).[3] Less commonly, hypernatremia is associated with increased sodium intake. This has been observed in animals eating beef jerky, home-made play dough, seawater, or iatrogenic administration of sodium-containing substances such as sodium bicarbonate or sodium phosphate enemas.[4]

Like hyponatremia, clinical signs associated with hypernatremia are usually nonspecific until hypernatremia becomes severe, and serum sodium exceeds 180 mEq/L. With acute elevations in serum sodium, water will move from an area of lower sodium concentration to an area of higher sodium concentration, and cells will shrink. Neuronal tissue is very sensitive to changes in intracellular volume, and reacts accordingly and adversely as serum sodium changes very rapidly. The clinical signs associated with severe acute hypernatremia are similar to those seen with hyponatremia, and include ataxia, depression, lethargy, stupor, coma, seizures, and in the most severe cases, death.

The goal of treating hypernatremia is to replace the free water deficit, in addition to treating primary cause, such as diarrhea. The rate at which serum sodium is normalized is directly proportional to the amount of time it took the patient to become hypernatremic. For example, in acute salt intoxication, the serum sodium concentration can be lowered more quickly than in an animal whose sodium has been gradually increasing over days to weeks. When serum sodium is so elevated that intracellular water moves into the extracellular space and causes cell shrinkage, the cells have an adaptive mechanism to combat cell shrinkage and decreased cell volume. Idiogenic osmoles are generated within the cells to help restore intracellular volume.[4] Idiogenic osmoles can be degraded when they are no longer needed, as serum sodium concentration is normalized. However, if serum sodium is treated too aggressively, in an attempt to normalize sodium concentration too rapidly, the intracellular compartment will be hyperosmolar with respect to the extracellular compartment, and fluid will rush into the cells, and cause cellular edema.

To treat hypernatremia, the free water deficit is calculated using the following formula:

$$\text{Free water deficit} = ([\text{current Na+}] \div [\text{normal Na}] - 1) \times (0.6 \times \text{kg body weight})$$

Ideally, serum sodium concentration should not be raised or lowered by more than 0.5 mEq/L per hour. In many cases, the administration of water with dextrose (D5W) is used to lower serum sodium. However, with severe hypernatremia, even 0.9% sodium chloride fluids contain a lot less sodium (154 mEq/L) than the patient's serum, and can be used for a gradual decrease, as tolerated.

Table 29
Causes of hypernatremia[2]

Diabetes insipidus
    Central (congenital or acquired)
        Neoplasia
        Trauma
        Pituitary malformation
        Inflammation
        Cysts
    Nephrogenic (congenital or acquired)
        Pyometra
        Hepatic disease
        Hyperadrenocorticism
        Hyperthyroidism
Free water loss
    Osmotic diarrhea
    Inadequate water intake
    Increased insensible fluid losses
    Heat stroke
    Vomiting
    Renal failure
Hyperaldosteronism
Ingestion of sodium
    Home-made play dough
    Seawater
    Meat jerky
Iatrogenic administration
    Sodium bicarbonate
    Sodium-containing enemas
    Table salt to induce emesis
Primary hypodipsia of Schnauzers

DISORDERS OF CHLORIDE

Chloride is the main anion in extracellular fluid, and is the predominant anion within the body.[3] Chloride, in addition to ions that dissociate within the body (strong ions), contributes to metabolic acidosis or alkalosis. Alterations in serum chloride are often dependent on the intravascular water or fluid volume status of the animal. As such, it is recommended to correct chloride concentration with respect to sodium. To correct chloride the following formulae are used:

Canines: Cl⁻ (corrected) = Cl⁻ × 146/Na
Felines: Cl⁻ (corrected) = Cl⁻ × 156/Na

Normally, the corrected values for chloride are 107–113 mEq/L in dogs and 117–123 mEq/L in cats.[3]

Hypochloremia

Hypochloremia is defined as a serum chloride concentration less than 100 mEq/L in dogs and less than 110 mEq/L in cats.[3] Potential causes of hypochloremia are listed in *Table 30*. Hypochloremia is a common electrolyte abnormality in animals with upper GI obstruction and vomiting gastric contents. Drugs can also induce hypochloremia by promoting renal or GI chloride loss.[3] In many cases, correction of the underlying condition and administration of intravenous fluids will correct hypochloremia.

Hyperchloremia

Hyperchloremia is defined as a serum chloride concentration above normal reference ranges. Causes of hyperchloremia are listed in *Table 31*. In many instances, the elevation in serum chloride concentration observed is artifactual, and is known as 'pseudohyperchloremia'. Conditions associated with free water loss, or loss of water in excess of choride loss, can be one cause. Other causes of pseudohyperchloremia include lipemic serum, the presence of hemoglobin or bilirubin pigment in serum, or potassium bromide administration.[3] Drugs and infusions such as parenteral nutrition can also result in elevations in serum chloride. Other causes of true hyperchloremia include renal failure, renal tubular acidosis, respiratory alkalosis, and diabetes mellitus.[3]

Table 30
Causes of hypochloremia

Pseudohypochloremia
    Hypoadrenocorticism
    Congestive heart failure
    Third-spacing of fluids (pleural or
    abdominal effusion)
True hypochloremia
    Upper GI obstruction with vomiting
    Loop diuretic administration
    Thiazide diuretic administration
    Sodium bicarbonate administration
    Carbenicillin administration
    Respiratory acidosis/hypercapnia (chronic)

Table 31
Causes of hyperchloremia

Artifactual hyperchloremia
    Diabetes insipidus
    Osmotic diuresis
    Lipemia
    Hemoglobinemia
    Bilirubinemia
    Potassium bromide administration
True hyperchloremia
    Drugs
        Potassium-sparing diuretic administration
            Spironolactone
            Amiloride
        Acetazolamide
        Parenteral nutrition
    Intravenous fluids
        Hypertonic saline
        0.9% sodium chloride
    Chloride salt administration
        Potassium chloride
        Magnesium chloride
        Calcium chloride
        Ammonium chloride
    Renal failure
    Renal tubular acidosis
    Repiratory alkalosis (chronic)
    Diabetes mellitus

DISORDERS OF POTASSIUM

Potassium is the most common cation in the body. The majority of potassium resides within cells, and a small amount (2–5%) is located in the extracellular space. The location and concentration of potassium within and outside the cells make it one of the most important ions within the body, as potassium plays a crucial role in enzymatic functions and metabolic processes, neuromuscular transmission, and muscular function. When potassium concentration is out of balance, whether it is too high or too low, neuromuscular deficits, including cardiac irritability and conduction defects, can become life-threatening.

Hypokalemia

Hypokalemia is a common electrolyte abnormality in critical illness. Causes of hypokalemia are listed in *Table 32*. The most common clinical manifestation of hypokalemia is muscular weakness. Animals may appear to walk stiffly, have cervical ventroflexion (**97**), adopt a plantigrade stance, and have generalized muscle weakness.[3,5] This is known as 'hypokalemic myopathy'.[6] Low serum potassium also has an

Table 32
Causes of hypokalemia[3]

Renal failure
Decreased potassium intake
Insulin administration
Vomiting
Diarrhea
Sodium bicarbonate administration
Hyperadrenocorticism
Polyuria
α-adrenergic drug administration or intoxication (albuterol)
Metabolic acidosis
Intravenous fluid diuresis
Hypothermia
Hypomagnesemia

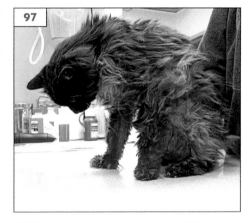

97 Cervical ventroflexion in a cat with severe hypokalemia. Another differential diagnosis in this patient is thiamine deficiency.

effect on cardiac conduction, with slowed repolarization and prolonged P-T interval and S-T segment depression.[5] T waves may have decreased amplitude, and various supraventricular and ventricular dysrhythmias may be present.

Treatment of hypokalemia involves treatment of the primary problem, when possible. For example, if hypokalemia has resulted from pyloric outflow obstruction, treatment of the vomiting, removal of the obstruction, and replenishing intravascular fluid volume with intravenous fluid and potassium supplementation is usually sufficient to correct the hypokalemia. Chronic renal failure is also a common cause of hypokalemia. Oral potassium supplementation can help restore serum potassium levels in such cases.

Hyperkalemia

Hyperkalemia is defined as serum potassium elevated above normal reference values. Causes of hyperkalemia are presented in *Table 33*. Hyperkalemia can result from decreased potassium excretion, increased potassium intake, or translocation of intracellular potassium to the extracellular space during conditions such as metabolic or diabetic ketoacidosis, or due to muscle breakdown and rhabdomyolysis.

Under normal conditions, aldosterone, secreted by the zona glomerulosa of the adrenal cortex, stimulates potassium excretion by the distal nephron. In animals with hypoadrenocorticism, who lack both cortisol and aldosterone, potassium excretion is blunted and results in hyperkalemia. Renal potassium excretion can also be impaired in conditions associated with oliguric or anuric renal failure. Oliguria or anuria can result from end-stage chronic renal failure, but are more commonly associated with urinary obstruction, renal ischemia, acute toxin, or bacterial infection (Lyme nephritis or leptospirosis, for example). Potassium can also become reabsorbed or not excreted in urethral obstruction or rupture of the ureters or urinary bladder.

The clinical consequences of elevated serum potassium become apparent in cardiac conductive tissue. As serum potassium becomes elevated, the charge gradient on either side of the cell membrane becomes diminished, i.e. the charge gradient essentially becomes more neutral, and diminishes the cell's capacity for depolarization. Atrial cells are particularly sensitive to the effects of hyperkalemia, and become refractory to depolarization. As serum potassium becomes higher and higher, characteristic changes on an electrocardiogram (ECG) include wide and spiked T waves, blunted, then smaller, prolonged P-R interval, and widened QRS complexes. Eventually, p

Table 33 Causes of hyperkalemia
Renal failure
Ruptured ureter, urinary bladder, urethra
Urinary obstruction
Hypoadrenocorticism
Trichuris vulpis infection
Third-spacing of fluids
Tissue trauma
Rhabdomyolysis
Pregnancy in Greyhounds
Hypoadrenocorticism
Acute tumor lysis syndrome
Crush injury
Drugs
Potassium-sparing diuretics
Angiotensin-converting enzyme inhibitors
Heparin
Succinylcholine

waves become absent, a condition known as atrial standstill (**98, 99**).

For any condition that results in clinically significant hyperkalemia, the two focal points of treatment are (1) to protect the heart from the myocardial effects of elevated serum potassium and (2) to treat the primary underlying cause of the hyperkalemia. Cardiac conduction abnormalities can be treated by two separate mechanisms. One mechanism is to drive the potassium intracellularly. This can be accomplished by administration of sodium bicarbonate (0.25–1 mEq/kg IV), or by administration of insulin (regular insulin, 0.25–0.5 units/kg IV) and dextrose (1 g dextrose IV per unit of insulin administered), followed by a constant rate infusion (2.5% IV). Sodium bicarbonate will create a temporary metabolic alkalosis. Intracellular hydrogen will exchange for potassium, so that the hydrogen ion can help neutralize the alkalosis. Potassium will be driven intracellularly. A second mechanism of treating hyperkalemia is to protect the myocardium from the toxic effects of the potassium. This is accomplished by introduction of another ion to raise the threshold of depolarization, namely calcium. Calcium can be administered in the form of calcium gluconate (0.5–1 mL/kg 10% IV slowly over 10 minutes) or calcium chloride (5–15 mg/kg/hr IV constant rate infusion [CRI]). Any of the therapies listed above usually take effect within 5 minutes and last for 40–60 minutes, while other therapies can be directed at treating the underlying cause of hyperkalemia. This author has frequently used a combination of insulin/dextrose and calcium gluconate.

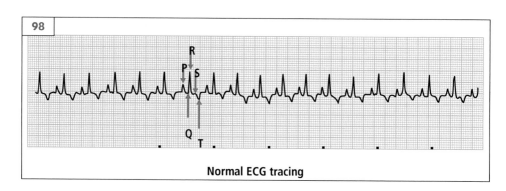

Normal ECG tracing

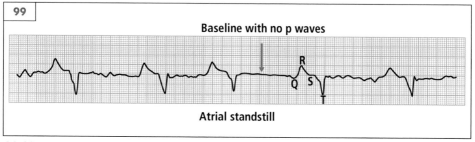

Baseline with no p waves

Atrial standstill

98 Normal ECG tracing, showing a p wave for every QRS, and a QRS for every p wave.
99 Atrial standstill in a patient with hyperkalemia. Note the absence of p waves on the baseline and the widened QRS complex and inverted, spiked T wave.

DISORDERS OF CALCIUM

The majority of the body's calcium is located within the hydroxyapatite matrix of bone. Only a small portion, roughly 1%, of calcium is located outside of the skeletal system in one of three forms: bound with protein, unionized, or ionized.[3] Ionized calcium is the biologically active form that is necessary for numerous enzymatic functions, coagulation, nervous system conduction, muscle contraction, and synthesis and production of new cells and cell membranes. Calcium concentration is regulated by a delicate balance of the active form of vitamin D (1-25, dihydroxycholecalciferol), parathyroid hormone synthesized and secreted by the parathyroid glands, the intestines, and the kidneys.

In the presence of ultraviolet light, the skin synthesizes fat-soluble vitamin D, or cholecalciferol. The parathyroid glands sense lower serum calcium concentration, and synthesize and produce parathyroid hormone. Parathyroid hormone (PTH) and vitamin D must both be present to increase calcium release from bone, and metabolism of vitamin D/cholecalciferol to its active form, calcitriol (1,25-dihydroxycholecalciferol). Calcitriol, in turn, functions to stimulate the absorption of calcium from the small intestine and the kidneys. Both hypo- and hypercalcemia are observed in a variety of clinical conditions, and can become life-threatening if left untreated.

Hypocalcemia

Clinically significant hypocalcemia can result in muscle irritability, tremors, hypotension, bradycardia, muscle weakness, panting, seizures, and cardiac or respiratory arrest. The most common causes of hypocalcemia in veterinary patients are associated with parathyroidectomy, renal disease, administration of blood transfusions and associated anticoagulants or drugs that chelate calcium, ethylene glycol toxicity, or puerperal tetany (eclampsia) (*Table 34*). Facial twitching is one of the first signs observed, and can progress to more severe muscle tremors, titanic spasms, and seizures. The treatment of clinically significant hypocalcemia involves the administration of calcium, in the form of either calcium gluconate (0.5–1.5 mL/kg 10% calcium gluconate IV slowly over 10 minutes) or calcium chloride (5–15 mg/kg/h IV CRI). In some cases a CRI of calcium gluconate (10 mg/kg/h IV CRI) may become necessary in hypocalcemic animals that are refractory to intermittent boluses of calcium gluconate or calcium chloride and oral calcitriol and oral calcium supplementation.

Table 34
Causes of hypocalcemia[3,7]

Disorders of parathyroid metabolism
    Primary hypoparathyroidism
    Iatrogenic after parathyroidectomy
    Iatrogenic after thyroidectomy
    Hypomagnesemia
Disorders of vitamin D metabolism
    Lack of activation of vitamin D in acute or chronic renal failure
    Intestinal malabsorption/malnutrition
    Anorexia
Eclampsia (puerperal tetany)
Pancreatitis (saponification)
Ethylene glycol intoxication
Chelation with citrated blood transfusion administration
Sodium bicarbonate therapy
Sodium phosphate enemas
Soft tissue trauma

Hypercalcemia

Hypercalcemia is defined as a total serum calcium concentration greater than 12 mg/dL (3 mmol/L) in dogs, and greater than 11 mg/dL (2.75 mmol/L) in cats.[3] As ionized calcium is the active form of calcium, ionized calcium should also be evaluated. Hypercalcemia is also defined as an ionized calcium greater than 5.2 mg/dL (1.3 mmol/L).[3] There are a number of mnemonics to aid in remembering the causes of hypercalcemia, listed in *Table 35*. When possible, treatment ideally should be directed at treating the underlying primary cause. Clinical signs related to hypercalcemia may involve the GI, renal, and neuromuscular systems. Polyuria, polydipsia, vomiting, anorexia, diarrhea, or constipation may be present.[3] A variety of cardiac rhythm disturbances, including ventricular dysrhythmias, prolonged PR interval, and short QT interval, may be observed on ECG. When the calcium × phosphorus product exceeds 70, dystrophic mineralization of soft tissues can occur in any organ. Treatment of hypercalcemia involves the administration of intravenous fluid diuresis with 0.9% saline to promote renal calciuresis, loop diuretics (furosemide 2–4 mg/kg IV q8–12h) to prevent renal calcium reabsorption, and glucocorticoids to inhibit bone reabsorption and activation of vitamin D.[3] In severe cases, drugs that promote calcium deposition, such as pamidronate or calcitonin, may be required to reduce serum calcium.

Table 35
Causes of hypercalcemia: GOSHDARNIT mnemonic[3,9]

Granulomatous
  Histoplasmosis
  Blastomycosis
  Cryptococcus
Osteogenic
Spurious
  Laboratory error
  Lipemia
  Hemolysis
Hyperparathyroidism
  Parathyroid adenoma
    Calcipotriene medication ingestion (psoriasis)
    Plant ingestion
      Cestrus diurnum
      Solanum malacoxylon
      Trisetum flavascens
D Vitamin D ingestion or cholecalciferol rodenticide toxicosis
Addison's disease
Renal failure
Neoplasia
  Lymphoma
  Apocrine gland adenocarcinoma
  Mammary adenocarcinoma
  Multiple myeloma
  Squamous cell carcinoma
Idiopathic
  Idiopathic hypercalcemia of cats
Temperature and toxicity
  Hyperthermia

DISORDERS OF PHOSPHORUS

Phosphorus is the most common intracellular ion.[3] The majority of phosphorus is located within the hydroxyapatite matrix of bone and in muscle.[3] A small amount of phosphorus is located in the extracellular space. Inorganic phosphate can be found bound to proteins such as albumin, and in circulation bound to hydrogen molecules. Inorganic phosphate can be measured in the serum. The other form of phosphate, organic phosphate, cannot be measured, and is an important component of cell membranes when bound with lipids and proteins. Organic phosphate is also used in the production of energy intermediates adenosine triphosphate (ATP) and adenosine diphosphate (ADP), and is involved in red blood cell oxygen delivery as 2,3-diphosphoglycerate (2,3-DPG).

Table 36
Causes of hypophosphatemia[3]

Redistribution
    Hyperventilation/respiratory alkalosis
    Refeeding syndrome
    Salicylate toxicosis
    Heat-induced illness/heat stroke
    Insulin administration
Decreased renal tubular uptake
Glucocorticoid administration
Diuretic administration
Sodium bicarbonate administration
Diabetes mellitus
Hyperadrenocorticism
Hyperaldosteronism
Hyperparathyroidism
Hypothermia
Parenteral nutrition administration
Gastrointestinal causes
    Decreased intake/anorexia
    Exocrine pancreatic insufficiency
    Deficiency of vitamin D
    Administration of phosphate binders
    Maldigestion/malabsorption

Hypophosphatemia

A list of conditions which can be associated with hypophosphatemia are shown in *Table 36*. Clinically significant hypophosphatemia occurs when serum inorganic phosphate levels drop below 1.0 mg/dL (0.32 mmol/L). The most common causes of hypophosphatemia in small animal patients are hyperventilation (respiratory alkalosis), diabetic ketoacidosis (DKA), and refeeding syndrome. In patients with DKA, renal excretion of phosphorus is increased due to glucosuria and osmotic diuresis. The administration of insulin during treatment of DKA can result in phosphorus moving intracellularly, and can cause a significant decrease in inorganic phosphate in the serum. When serum phosphate levels drop to less than 1.0 mg/dL (0.32 mmol/L), red cell hemolysis (**100**) and anemia can result. In animals with severe long-term anorexia and malnourishment, rapid administration of the patient's full caloric requirements can cause a massive release of insulin from the pancreas, and cause the movement of phosphate from the extracellular to the intracellular space. Additionally, whole body depletion of phosphate during times of starvation, then the utilization of available phosphate to form ADP and ATP, cause further depletion of inorganic phosphate and can also result in cardiac conduction abnormalities, muscle weakness, and RBC hemolysis. The treatment of clinically significant hypophosphatemia involves phosphorus supplementation in the form of potassium or sodium phosphate (0.03–0.06 mmol/kg/h IV CRI for 12–24 hours). Some clinicians empirically treat patients with DKA with phosphorus supplementation as a general part of treatment, to avoid complications associated with hypophosphatemia.

Hyperphosphatemia

Hyperphosphatemia is less commonly observed in veterinary patients than hypophosphatemia. A list of possible causes of hyperphosphatemia is shown in *Table 37*. The most common causes of hyperphosphatemia are renal insufficiency, GI inflammation, and GI hemorrhage. When seen in combination with hypercalcemia, a calcium × phosphorus product greater than 70 can result in dystrophic mineralization of soft tissues. Other clinical signs of hyperphosphatemia include diarrhea and tetanic muscle spasms. The treatment of hyperphosphatemia includes treatment of the primary disorder and prevention of phosphorus absorption from the GI tract. If an animal is eating, restriction of dietary phosphorus intake in addition to oral phosphate binders such as aluminum hydroxide can reduce small intestinal phosphorus absorption.

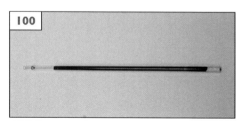

100 Intravascular hemolysis, with red-colored plasma in the hematocrit tube, from a patient with severe hypophosphatemia. Although this condition is more commonly observed following treatment of diabetic ketoacidosis with insulin, it can also be observed in animals with refeeding syndrome.

Table 37
Causes of hyperphosphatemia

Renal failure
Hemolysis
Acute tumor lysis syndrome
Rhabdomyolysis
Soft tissue injury
Sodium phosphate enemas
Hypoparathyroidism
Acromegaly
Vitamin D toxicosis

DISORDERS OF MAGNESIUM

Magnesium is one of the most important, and often forgotten, intracellular cations. The majority of the body's magnesium is located within bone and muscle tissue. A very small amount of magnesium is located within the extracellular space. One of the most important functions of magnesium is as a cofactor for the Na–K–ATPase pump that maintains the electrochemical gradient across cell membranes of excitable tissue. Magnesium is also required as a cofactor in the production of cellular ATP. Thus magnesium is extremely important in the health and well-being of veterinary patients.

Like calcium, magnesium exists in three forms: ionized, complexed with other substances, and bound to protein. It is very difficult to measure magnesium, because the majority of it is located in intracellular stores. Measurement of serum magnesium, therefore, does not necessarily reflect total body magnesium, or intracellular magnesium available for metabolic and enzymatic processes.

Hypomagnesemia

Hypomagnesemia has been reported to be present in 54–67% of critically ill veterinary patients,[8,9] and is commonly found in association with other electrolyte abnormalities, which include hyponatremia, hypokalemia, hypocalcemia, and hypophosphatemia (*Table 38*).[3] As magnesium is required for the Na–K–ATPase pump that helps maintain

Table 38
Causes of hypomagnesemia[3,7]

Decreased magnesium intake	**Digoxin**
Malnourishment	**Diuretics**
Anorexia	Loop diuretics (furosemide)
Iatrogenic administration of fluids without	Osmotic diuretics (mannitol)
magnesium	Thiazide diuretics
Gastrointestinal	**Endocrinopathies**
Diarrhea	Diabetic ketoacidosis
Malabsorption/maldigestion	Hyperadrenocorticism
Exocrine pancreatic insufficiency	Hyperthyroidism
Short bowel syndrome after bowel	Hyperparathyroidism
resection	Hypercalcemia
Inflammatory bowel disease	Hypophosphatemia
Renal	**Respiratory alkalosis**
Acute renal failure	**Pancreatitis**
Renal tubular acidosis	**Peritoneal dialysis**
Glomerulonephritis	**Blood transfusion**
Pyelonephritis	**Insulin and/or dextrose administration**
Post-obstructive diuresis	**Trauma**
Drugs	**Sepsis**
Amphotericin B	**Burns**
Aminoglycosides	**Shearing injuries**
Carbenicillin	**Hypothermia**
Ciclosporin	

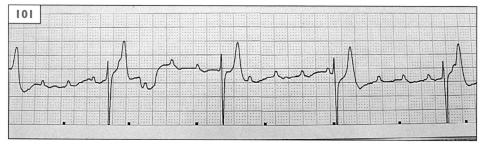

101 Complete atrioventricular block. Note that there are multiple p waves in complete dissociation with the intermittent ventricular escape beats.

sodium and potassium concentrations, deficiencies in magnesium can lead to hypokalemia and kaliuresis. This is commonly observed in hypokalemic patients with diabetic ketoacidosis who are treated with very high rates of potassium supplementation, and appear refractory to therapy. Other clinical signs of hypomagnesemia include cardiac conduction abnormalities and refractory supraventricular and ventricular dysrhythmias, weakness, muscle tremors, and progressive neurologic dysfunction which includes hypoventilation, dysphagia, seizures, coma, and respiratory muscle fatigue.[3] Supplementation of magnesium (magnesium chloride 0.75 mEq/kg/day IV CRI) often quickly results in normalization of the previously refractory hypokalemia. Overzealous supplementation of magnesium can result in cardiac rhythm disturbances, including bundle branch and atrioventricular block (**101**). Magnesium supplementation should be carefully titrated, and used with caution in animals with renal insufficiency.

Hypermagnesemia

Hypermagnesemia is fairly uncommon in critically ill veterinary patients, but when present is associated with an increased risk of mortality (*Table 39*).[8] Magnesium is excreted by the kidneys. Hypermagnesemia can occur in animals with oliguric or anuric renal failure due to lack of magnesium excretion. In cases of severe hypermagnesemia, cardiac conduction abnormalities including prolonged PR interval and widened QRS complexes, neuromuscular weakness, and respiratory muscle fatigue may be observed. Treatment of hypermagnesemia is aimed primarily at increasing renal magnesium excretion with the use of 0.9% sodium chloride intravenous fluid diuresis and the administration of loop diuretics such as furosemide.

Table 39
Causes of hypermagnesemia[3]

Iatrogenic administration of magnesium-containing salts or fluids

Renal insufficiency/failure

Magnesium antacid administration/ingestion

Magnesium salt cathartics

Parenteral nutrition

- **Introduction**

- **Parenteral nutrition**

- **Complications of parenteral nutrition**

- **Conclusions**

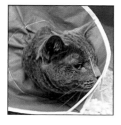
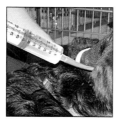
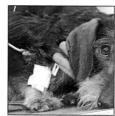

INTRODUCTION

Iatrogenic malnourishment, or inadequate nutrient intake during hospitalization, is unfortunately a too common occurrence in veterinary patients.[1] Many hospitalized patients either will not eat voluntarily, or have illnesses referrable to the GI tract, such as vomiting and/or diarrhea, that prevent them from digesting, absorbing, or assimilating the nutrients that are fed to them. A common and easily reparable problem is that vague food orders are prescribed by the attending clinician. Decreased intake of calories, protein, and other essential nutrients can contribute to increased patient morbidity, depressed or delayed wound healing, suppression of the immune system, and possibly increased patient mortality.

In more recent years, knowledge of the consequences of malnutrition and advances in the ability to provide enteral and parenteral nutrition to veterinary patients has allowed practitioners not only to become more aggressive when feeding hospitalized patients, but also has empowered clinicians to be well-informed and less tolerant of iatrogenic malnutrition in critically ill small animal patients. The goals of nutritional support are to treat and prevent malnutrition during times of critical illness until the patient is able to assimilate enteral nutrients alone.[2] Provision of some form of enteral nutrition is considered to be the gold standard for nutritional support. (**102**) Whatever portion of the GI tract is functional should be utilized. However, some animals either cannot or will not eat voluntarily, or cannot digest or absorb the nutrients that are provided enterally due to severe vomiting, ileus, inflammation, or surgical resection of the GI tract.[2,3] In such cases, enteral nutrition may be contraindicated or not possible, and other forms of nutritional support, such as parenteral nutrition (**103**), becomes absolutely necessary.

Parenteral nutrition provides nutrients by a method other than the GI tract.[4] Ideal mixtures of nutrients for parenteral nutrition include a carbohydrate solution, usually in the form of dextrose, a lipid, an amino acid or protein source, and in some cases, minerals and vitamins (*Table 40*).

The term 'total parenteral nutrition' or TPN, is used to describe the solution used to provide all of a patient's essential nutrient requirements.[5,6] In veterinary patients, however, every single essential macro- and micronutrient is rarely provided. For this reason, the term TPN is actually a misnomer that is now discouraged from use.[4] A more accurate term is 'partial parenteral nutrition' (PPN) or simply parenteral nutrition (PN).[6]

Some individuals characterize and identify PN based on its route of administration. Solutions that have an osmolality greater than 600 mOsm/L should ideally be infused through a central venous or intraosseous catheter, to avoid the potential complication of thrombophlebitis.[7] If the osmolality is less than 600 mOsm/L, the solution can be infused through a peripheral catheter, with low potential to cause thrombophlebitis. When the solution is infused through a peripheral catheter, the term 'peripheral parenteral nutrition' has been suggested. Peripheral parenteral nutrition should be considered only when the nutritional support is required for a brief period of time, such as 1–3 days. If an animal needs nutritional supplementation for a longer period of time, careful assessment of the benefits of placing a central venous catheter for administration of a more complete nutrient admixture, or placement of some form of enteral feeding tube, should be considered. Peripheral parenteral nutrition is also used when an animal is voluntarily ingesting only a portion of its daily nutrient intake, and still needs some nutritional support via parenteral means.

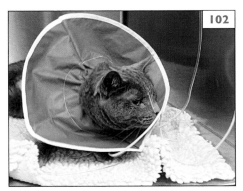

102 Nasoesopharyngeal tube feeding in a cat with hepatic lipidosis.

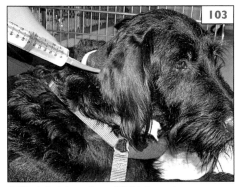

103 Administration of fluid through an esophagostomy tube in a patient with acute renal failure secondary to ingestion of food that had been contaminated with melamine.

Table 40
Parenteral nutrition components

Name	Osmolality (mOsm/L)	pH	Manufacturer
10% Amino acid (Travasol)	998	6.0	Baxter Healthcare Corporation (UK and Canada)
8.5% Aminosyn	850	4.5–6.0	Abbott Pharmaceuticals
Procalamine	735	6.8	McGaw, Inc.
5% Dextrose	252–310	3.2–6.5	Abbott Pharmaceuticals
50% Dextrose	2530	4.2	Abbott Pharmaceuticals
20% Amino acid (Aminosyn)	260	8.3	Abbott Pharmaceuticals
Intralipid 20%	350	6.0–8.9	Baxter Healthcare Corporation (UK and Canada)
Intralipid 20%	350	6.0–8.9	Fresenius Kabi
2% Liposyn			Abbott Pharmaceuticals

Central catheter placement

Infusion of a hyperosmolar substance into a peripheral vein is often associated with the development of thrombophlebitis. It is recommended, therefore, that PN solutions with an osmolality greater than 600 mOsm/L should be infused into a central venous catheter. In small animal patients, central venous catheters can be placed into the jugular, medial saphenous, and lateral saphenous veins with relative ease. A number of single- and multiple-lumen catheter types are available. Polyurethane and silicone catheters have been shown to be less irritating to the vessels, and have been recommended over Teflon catheters.[6] One of the most important concepts to remember when placing a central venous catheter is to maintain sterility at all times, in order to prevent catheter-related sepsis. Once the catheter has been successfully placed and bandaged, the PN solution can be connected. The line should be labeled as a dedicated line, and not be used for any other purpose other than administration of the nutritional support. The line should not be disconnected for any reason except to change fluid/nutrition bags every 24 hours, even when taking the patient for a walk outside. The bandage should be changed and the catheter entrance site examined every 24 hours. Signs of phlebitis include erythema and pain at the catheter site, pain upon infusion into the vessel, and ropiness or hardening of the vessel on external palpation. In several retrospective studies on the use of central venous catheters for infusion of PN, catheter occlusion and kinking were among the most common complications observed.[8–10]

PARENTERAL NUTRITION

In the past, high expense, perceived fear of catheter-related sepsis, and lack of technical expertise and supplies required for administration of parenteral nutrition made this mode of nutritional support uncommon in veterinary medicine.[7,11] Placement of central venous and multi-lumen central catheters has become more common in veterinary patients, making the possibility of providing PN easier.[11] Advances in the understanding of aseptic technique when placing and then maintaining central venous catheters can limit the incidence of catheter-related sepsis. If sepsis occurs in a patient on PN, the origin of the bacterial infection is often not the catheter itself. Rather, the enterocytes that line the GI tract start to atrophy within 48 hours of lack of enteral nutrition. Tight junctions in the basement membrane open and become leaky, and provide a means for bacteria to translocate from the GI tract into the bloodstream.

Parenteral nutrition formulation

The components of a PN solution can be either mixed at a compounding pharmacy, or mixed in-house. Essential components of any PN solution include amino acids, dextrose, lipid, vitamins, and minerals. Ideally, the solutions should be prepared under strict aseptic conditions, in a laminar-flow hood or in a specialized compounding machine.[7] One such device is sold in the UK by Baxter, and is called 'The Automix'. Compounding machines can be used to formulate accurate PN solutions under sterile conditions. 'Three-in-one' mixtures are also available that contain an amino acid, lipid, and dextrose source. The prefabricated PN formulations that are available from some veterinary and human manufacturers (e.g. Abbott Animal Health) are meant to make provision of PN for patients easier, and more accessible for the veterinary practitioner. Although this type of product is more efficient for use, as it does not require specialized compounding equipment, whenever possible the PN solution should be formulated based on the individual patient's needs, rather than using a mixture that may over- or underestimate the caloric and protein needs of a particular animal. Pharmacies in a local human hospital can be solicited to help mix PN for the small animal patient.

The resting energy expenditure (REE) is the amount of calories required by an animal that is resting, in a thermoneutral environment, in a post-prandial state. These criteria rarely describe a hospitalized animal with some form of critical illness that requires nutritional support. It is, however, the closest approximation available to estimate the patients' caloric requirements (*Table 41*). In the past, the caloric requirements of animals were largely extrapolated from human literature or from data obtained from healthy dogs and cats. The REE was then arbitrarily multiplied by an 'illness, injury, infection/inflammation' factor, with the presumption that animals with illness or other conditions have higher than normal energy demands. This recommendation has been abandoned in recent years, when the results of research conducted in veterinary critical care

units showed that critically ill small animal patients actually require basal energy requirements,[12] and are not 'hypermetabolic' as previously suggested. In fact, the caloric requirements of an individual animal can change from day to day throughout the course of hospitalization.[13]

A linear equation to calculate a patient's daily caloric requirements or REE is:

$$REE = (30 \times \text{body weight}_{kg}) + 70 = \text{kcal/day}$$

This may potentially underestimate the caloric needs of some animals and overestimate the needs of others (*Table 41*). Oversupplementation of carbohydrates, in particular, can lead to an increase in respiratory work owing to the need to eliminate excess CO_2 created as a byproduct of carbohydrate metabolism.

Once an animal's daily energy requirements (REE) have been calculated, the next component to consider is what percentage of the REE will be administered in the form of

Table 41
Resting energy expenditure (REE)

Body weight in lb	Weight in kg	Daily REE (kcal)	Maintenance +7%	Maintenance +10%	Maintenance +12%
2.2	1	96	170	200	220
4.4	2	120	270	330	370
6.6	3	168	370	460	520
8.8	4	192	470	590	670
11.0	5	216	570	720	820
13.2	6	240	670	850	970
15.4	7	288	770	980	1120
17.6	8	312	870	1110	1270
19.8	9	336	970	1240	1420
22.0	10	360	1070	1370	1570
24.2	11	408	1170	1500	1720
26.4	12	432	1270	1630	1870

(*Continued*)

Table 41
Resting energy expenditure (REE) (*Continued*)

Body weight in lb	Weight in kg	Daily REE (kcal)	Maintenance +7%	Maintenance +10%	Maintenance +12%
28.6	13	456	1370	1760	2020
30.8	14	480	1470	1890	2170
33.0	15	528	1570	2020	2320
35.2	16	552	1670	2150	2470
37.4	17	576	1770	2280	2620
39.6	18	600	1870	2410	2770
41.8	19	648	1970	2540	2920
44.0	20	672	2070	2670	3070
46.2	21	696	2170	2800	3220
48.4	22	720	2270	2930	3370
50.6	23	768	2370	3060	3520
52.8	24	792	2470	3190	3670
55.0	25	816	2570	3320	3820
57.2	26	840	2670	3450	3970
59.4	27	888	2770	3580	4120
61.6	28	912	2870	3710	4270
63.8	29	936	2970	3840	4420
66.0	30	960	3070	3970	4570
70.4	32	1032	3270	4230	4870
74.8	34	1080	3470	4490	5170
79.2	36	1152	3670	4750	5470
83.6	38	1200	3870	5010	5770
88.0	40	1272	4070	5270	6070
92.4	42	1320	4270	5530	6370
96.8	44	1392	4470	5790	6670
101.2	46	1440	4670	6050	6970
105.6	48	1512	4870	6310	7270
110.0	50	1560	5070	6570	7570
114.4	52	1632	5270	6830	7870
118.8	54	1680	5470	7090	8170
123.2	56	1752	5670	7350	8470
127.6	58	1800	5870	7610	8770
132.0	60	1872	6070	7870	9070
143.0	65	2016	6570	8520	9820
154.0	70	2160	7070	9170	10570
165.0	75	2328	7570	9820	11320
176.0	80	2472	8070	10470	12070
187.0	85	2616	8570	11120	12820
198.0	90	2760	9070	11770	13570
209.0	95	2928	9570	12420	14320
220.0	100	3072	10070	13070	15070

carbohydrate, and what percentage will be administered as lipid. In general, 20% of the REE is provided by dextrose, and 80% of the REE provided as lipid.[6] The amount of protein to administer can be calculated from the REE relative to the amount of nonprotein calories required by the individual patient. Protein requirements range from 1–6 g protein/100 kcal nonprotein energy in small animal patients.[6] In dogs, approximately 2–3 g of protein/100 kcal nonprotein calories should be administered on a daily basis. In cats, the value is slightly higher, at 4 g protein/100 kcal.[6] In animals with hepatic or renal insufficiency, smaller amounts of protein should be administered; in patients with large amounts of protein loss, larger portions should be considered. Long-term management of veterinary patients with PN for more than a couple of weeks is extremely uncommon. In the rare instance that long-term PN is required, one

must consider that most amino acid solutions do not contain the essential amino acid taurine. Additional supplementation with this amino acid should be considered if a cat is on PN for more than 7 days.

The concentrations of lipid, dextrose, and amino acid in each component solution, and the calories per milliliter of the lipid and dextrose solutions, influence the volumes to be added to the PN solution. Once the volume of each component (amino acid + lipid + dextrose) has been calculated, the total volume is added together, then the sum is divided by 24, to obtain the rate in mL/hour. An example of a step-by-step calculation of PN is presented in *Table 42*. A bag of PN can be refrigerated for up to 48 hours. Once the bag is at room temperature, however, it should be administered within 24 hours, then discarded.

Table 42
Step-wise approach to calculating parenteral nutrition formulation

1. Calculate the patient's daily resting energy requirement (REE in kcal/day):

   $$REE = (30 \times BW_{kg}) + 70$$

2. Calculate the patient's carbohydrate source, providing 20% of REE as dextrose.
3. Calculate the patient's lipid requirement, providing 80% of REE as lipid.
4. Calculate the patient's daily amino acid (protein) requirement (3 g/100 kcal for dogs, and 4 g/100 kcal for cats).
5. Use the following guidelines to determine the volume of each parenteral nutrition component required:

   5% dextrose = 0.17 kcal/mL
   50% dextrose = 1.7 kcal/mL
   20% lipid = 2 kcal/mL
   8.5% amino acid (protein) = 0.085 g/mL
   3% amino acid (protein) = 0.03 g/mL

(*Continued*)

Table 42
Step-wise approach to calculating parenteral nutrition formulation (*Continued*)

6. Add the volume of dextrose, lipid, and amino acid (protein) solution together to yield a daily volume to be administered.
7. Divide the volume obtained in Step 6 by 24 hours, to yield a mL/hour rate of infusion.
    OR
8. Determine the patient's daily fluid requirement.
9. Subtract the volume obtained in Step 6 from the volume obtained in Step 8.
10. Add the volume obtained in Step 9 as an isotonic solution to the parenteral nutrition (components total volume in Step 6) to obtain a daily fluid and nutrition solution.
11. Divide the total volume of Step 10 by 24 hours, to yield a fluid rate per hour.

Example of calculating parenteral nutrition for a 30 kg dog:
1. Calculate the patient's daily REE:
    $(30 \times 30) + 70 = 970$ kcal/day
2. Calculate the daily carbohydrate source:
    $20\% = 0.2 \times 970$ kcal/day $= 194$ kcal/day carbohydrate (dextrose)
3. Calculate the daily lipid source:
    $80\% = 0.8 \times 970$ kcal/day $= 776$ kcal/day lipid
4. Calculate the daily amino acid (protein) requirement (3 g amino acid [protein]/100 kcal in dogs):
    970 kcal/day $\times$ 3 g amino acid (protein)/100 kcal $= 29.1$ g amino acid (protein)/day
5. 50% dextrose $= 1.7$ kcal/mL:
    194 kcal $\times$ 1 mL/1.7 kcal $= 114$ mL of 50% dextrose/day
    20% lipid $= 2$ kcal/mL:
    776 kcal $\times$ 1 mL/2 kcal $= 388$ mL 20% lipid
    29.1 g amino acid (protein)/day $\times$ 1 mL/0.085 g amino acid (protein) $= 342$ mL/day 8.5% amino acid (protein)
6. Add the volume of dextrose, lipid, and amino acid (protein) required:
    114 mL 50% dextrose
    388 mL 20% lipid
    + 342 mL 8.5% amino acid (protein) $= 844$ mL/day
7. Divide the above volume by 24 to yield mL/hour rate of administration:
    844 mL/day $\div$ 24 hours $= 35.1 \approx 35$ mL/hour
    OR
8. Determine the patient's daily fluid requirement (60 mL/kg/day)
    60 mL/kg/day $\times$ 30 kg $= 1800$ mL/day
9. Subtract the parenteral nutrition volume from daily fluid requirement:
    1800 mL/day $-$ 844 mL/day $= 956$ mL
10. Add 956 mL of an isotonic fluid such as Normosol-R to the parenteral nutrition solution.
11. 1800 mL $\div$ 24 hours $= 75$ mL/hour of total nutrient admixture.

Amino acid solutions

Solutions of essential and nonessential crystalline amino acids (3.5%, 8.5%, and 15%) are available as a source of protein for veterinary PN use. An 8.5–10% amino acid solution (10% Travasol Amino Acid with and without electrolytes, Baxter UK and Baxter Canada; 8.5% Aminosyn Abbott Animal Health, USA) is used very commonly, as solutions with lower concentrations of amino acids require too large a volume of fluid to administer, and solutions with higher concentrations are extremely hyperosmolar.[6] The osmolality of amino acid solutions ranges from 300 mOsm/L to 1400 mOsm/L, and is relatively acidic, with a pH of 5.3–6.5.[6,14,15] Because of their hyperosmolality, amino acid solutions that are greater than 3.5% should not be administered through a peripheral venous catheter, owing to the high risk of thrombophlebitis.[15]

Lipids

Emulsions of soybean, safflower oil, linoleic acid, and linolenic acid are available as 10% and 20% lipid solutions in an isotonic fluid (Intralipid 20 or 30% soybean oil fat emulsion, Baxter Canada, Baxter UK, Intralipid 20% Fresenius Kabi in Europe, 20% Liposyn, Abbott Animal Health, USA).[6] Lipids are used to provide a minimum of 40–60% of an animal's daily nonprotein caloric requirements.[16] The osmolality of lipid emulsions (260–310 mOsm/L) is lower than that of amino acid solutions, and can be administered through a peripheral venous catheter without an increased risk of thrombophlebitis.[6,14,15]

Dextrose

Varying concentrations of dextrose (2.5–70%) are available as a carbohydrate source for PN formulations. A 50% dextrose solution is available to most veterinary practitioners and is mixed with the lipid and amino acid solutions to provide an animal's daily nutritional needs. The exact ratio of dextrose to lipid to meet a patient's caloric requirements is a topic of debate. During states of stressed starvation, glucocounter-regulatory hormones such as cortisol and epinephrine promote a state of insulin resistance. The body is unable to utilize carbohydrate sources for energy, and hyperglycemia can develop. In humans, hyperglycemia secondary to oversupplementation of carbohydrates has been shown to increase patient morbidity, respiratory failure by increasing respiratory work, and mortality. A similar study in cats documented an increased risk of mortality when hyperglycemia occurred during the course of PN administration.[10] In small animal patients, dextrose as provided in PN formulations should not exceed 50% of total daily caloric requirements.

Electrolytes

Electrolyte abnormalities are a common complication during the administration of PN in a critically ill animal. Hypokalemia and hypophosphatemia are among the most common electrolyte abnormalities observed. In animals that have had prolonged malnourishment, the administration of a dextrose-containing fluid can stimulate a massive amount of insulin to be released from the pancreas. This effect serves to drive glucose, potassium, and phosphorus intracellularly. Additionally, the production of energy intermediates such as ATP can also deplete phosphorus, leading to hypophosphatemia. Phosphorus is required for maintenance of RBC membrane integrity. Severe hypophosphatemia can result in intravascular hemolysis and anemia if not monitored and supplemented, when necessary. The monitoring of a patient's serum potassium and phosphorus is necessary in order to determine the appropriate amount of potassium and phosphorus supplementation. In most cases, adding 20–40 mEq/L of potassium chloride, or a mixture of potassium chloride with potassium phosphate (0.01–0.03 mmol/kg/hr), may be necessary to maintain normokalemia and normophosphatemia.[15]

Vitamins

Unless anorexia and weight loss have been very prolonged, most patients do not require supplementation with fat- and water-soluble vitamins. Vitamin supplementation may also be necessary if nutrient absorption has been diminished due to excessive diarrhea or steatorrhea.[6] A weekly dose of vitamin K1 (0.5 mg/kg subcutaneously) at the onset of parenteral nutrition has been suggested.[2,6] Repository solutions of other fat-soluble vitamins (A, D, and E; 1 mL IM, Schering-Plough Animal Healthcorp, Kenilworth, NJ) are also available, and will provide a sufficient store for approximately 3 months.[6] B-complex vitamins can be provided as a combination preparation in the PN (1 mL/100 kcal or 3 mL/10 kg/day).[2] Because some B vitamins degrade when exposed to light, the PN solution should be covered to prevent degradation of labile substances.

Total nutrient admixture

Parenteral nutrition solutions need to be administered through a designated line, or a designated port if a multi-lumen catheter has been placed. In some instances, it may be difficult to obtain vascular access in a peripheral vein for the provision of crystalloid fluids. The practice of 'piggy-backing' one solution onto another by inserting a needle into a port somewhere in the intravenous fluid line is discouraged because of the risk of bacterial contamination of the fluid line.

A simple method of providing the patient's total daily nutritional and fluid requirements is to combine the PN in a lactated Ringer's or other isotonic fluid (e.g. Normosol-R, Plasmalyte-A) bag. First, the volume of each PN component is determined. Next, the patient's total daily fluid requirement is determined. The volume of the PN is adjusted to meet the patient's daily fluid requirements by adding an isotonic fluid such as lactated Ringer's, Plasmalyte-A or -148, or Normosol-R into the bag of PN. However, since the REE and hence fluid requirements do not take into account rehydration estimates or ongoing fluid losses, the fluid requirements often need to be adjusted to meet the individual patient's needs, and are often greater than the REE and fluid volume provided as PN.

The additions of fluids into the PN formulation, or *vice versa*, should be made aseptically, and the resultant fluid infused into a dedicated line. The advantage of administering a total nutrient admixture solution is that the patient requires just one dedicated catheter, one fluid administration set, and one fluid pump.[4]

Partial parenteral nutrition

PPN is the provision of a portion of a patient's daily nutritional requirements. PPN should be used only in cases where nutritional support is anticipated for less than 5 days, or during a transition period when a patient is consuming only a portion of their daily nutritional requirements enterally. The osmolality of PPN formulations is usually lower than 600 mOsm/L, and therefore they can be administered through a peripheral vein. Since amino acid solutions are very hyperosmolar, peripheral parenteral solutions typically contain small amounts of amino acid, and provide a portion of the patient's caloric requirements as a mixture of dextrose and iso-osmolar lipid solutions. Because of volume and osmolality constraints, PPN only provides a portion of a patient's daily nutrient needs.[13,17]

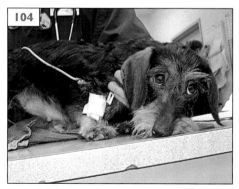

104 Administration of parenteral nutrition through a jugular central venous catheter in a Dachshund with pancreatitis.

COMPLICATIONS OF PARENTERAL NUTRITION

Nutrition is one of the most important aspects of therapy in a critically ill or injured patient. Enteral nutrition is preferred, whenever possible, but in some cases, PN must be administered owing to enteral feeding intolerance or a malfunctioning GI tract. One of the most common reasons for not implementing PN support in critically ill veterinary patients is the perception of numerous complications. Several studies have been published investigating the use of PN in veterinary patients. Complications associated with PN administration can be categorized as mechanical, septic, or metabolic.[3,8] Mechanical complications are most common, and are typically associated with catheter dislodgement, kinks, and clogging.[3,8–10] Many PN products are hyperosmolar, and can contribute to thrombophlebitis. As a general rule, PN solutions whose osmolality is less than 600 mOsm/L can be administered short-term though a peripheral venous catheter, but solutions greater than 600 mOsm/L should be administered through a central venous catheter. Perivascular administration of dextrose-containing fluids, including PN, can cause erythema and pain.

In several veterinary studies, septic complications during administration of parenteral nutrition were few and were associated with the patient's primary disease process, or due to disruption of the patient's designated infusion line.[3,8–10] Catheter-related sepsis can occur, particularly with disconnection of the fluid line, and sampling of blood products or infusion of drugs through a catheter used for PN. Guidelines to avoid the potential for catheter-induced sepsis include not disconnecting the PN fluid line, designating the catheter and line specifically for the sole purpose of PN, and changing the PN fluid line every 24 hours, or if it becomes contaminated. Lack of enteral nutrition can promote disuse atrophy of enterocytes and promote bacterial translocation and sepsis. Administration of even very small amounts (1–3 mL/kg/hr, or 'trickle feeding') of enteral nutrition in the form of a balanced commercially available product or amino acid solution can reduce the risk of enterocyte atrophy, even if the patient is vomiting.[18]

Metabolic complications include transient hyperglycemia, hypokalemia, hyperlipidemia, hypophosphatemia, hyperbilirubinemia, hyponatremia, and hypochloremia.[3,8–10] In one study[9], hyperglycemia at 24 hours after onset of PN infusion was associated with increased risk of mortality. In human patients, persistent hyperglycemia can contribute to respiratory fatigue and increased patient mortality. Administration of 10 units of regular insulin per liter of PN can reduce the hyperglycemia associated with PN administration.[3] Careful monitoring of the PN catheter and catheter site, as well as acid–base, electrolyte, and glucose monitoring, should be performed at least once a day to avoid these potential complications.

Refeeding syndrome can occur when an animal has been inappetant for long periods of time, then fed its minimum caloric requirements or more. Refeeding syndrome potentially can be difficult to treat or deadly. Administration of enteral or parenteral nutrition to severely malnourished animals provides the building blocks for energy production, namely the production of ATP. The carbohydrate sources administered in parenteral or enteral nutrition products will stimulate the release of insulin from the pancreas. Insulin will promote the shift of potassium and phosphorus into the intracellular space. Further, as ATP is produced, phosphorus stores can become depleted. Severe hypophosphatemia can result in intravascular hemolysis and anemia, sometimes requiring blood cell transfusion. Whenever parenteral (or enteral) nutrition is administered to an animal that has been anorexic for more than several days, a general rule is to provide only one-third of its resting energy requirements on the first day, then gradually increase the amount of calories provided over 3–4 days. Ideally, serum phosphorus should be evaluated twice daily initially, to ensure hypophosphatemia is not occurring. Electrolytes should be monitored at least twice daily along with packed cell volume (PCV) and total solids (TS). Blood glucose can be monitored every 2–8 hours as necessary, to ensure hypo- or severe hyperglycemia is not occurring.

CONCLUSIONS

PN should be considered in any patient that cannot tolerate enteral feeding. Nutritional plans should be formulated based on individual patient requirements, disease processes, anticipated duration of required nutritional support, and risk of complications. Even while the animal is receiving PN, daily reassessment of the need for PN is necessary. Enteral nutrition should always be offered, so that if and when the patient develops an appetite, food is available for ingestion. As the amount of enteral feeding increases, parenteral feeding can be gradually reduced. The risk of increased patient morbidity and mortality and delayed wound healing greatly exceeds the perceived risks of increased patient expense and mechanical, metabolic, or septic complications. With increased use and technical proficiency, placement of dedicated central venous catheters and administration of PN can become commonplace in all veterinary hospitals, provided that aseptic techniques are strictly adhered to.

CHAPTER 8

Shock: recognition, pathophysiology, monitoring, and treatment

- **Introduction**

- **Hypovolemic shock**

- **Cardiogenic shock**

- **Distributive shock**

- **Obstructive shock**

- **Care and 'Rule of Twenty'**

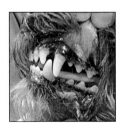
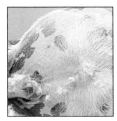
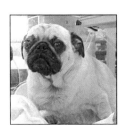
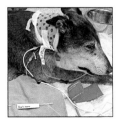

INTRODUCTION

Shock is defined as a condition in which there is inadequate effective circulating blood flow to meet cellular oxygen demands.[1] There are various forms of shock, which differ in the underlying mechanisms by which there is impaired tissue oxygen delivery (*Table 43*). In this chapter, the clinical signs, pathophysiology, recognition, monitoring, and treatment of various shock states will be discussed.

HYPOVOLEMIC SHOCK

Hypovolemia is a state of decreased circulating intravascular fluid volume.[2,3] Hypovolemia can be associated with the most severe forms of dehydration secondary to vomiting or diarrhea, but more commonly is associated with intravascular fluid loss from internal or external hemorrhage or wound exudates. A state of relative hypovolemia occurs when the vascular beds dilate inappropriately or in response to vasodilatory agents such as gas anesthetics.

Table 43
Causes of shock

Hypovolemic	**Cardiogenic**
Hemorrhage	Mitral regurgitation
Trauma	Bacterial endocarditis
Neoplasia	Tricuspid regurgitation
Coagulation disorders	Dilative cardiomyopathy
Extreme dehydration	Hypertrophic cardiomyopathy
Vomiting	Restrictive or unclassified cardiomyopathy
Diarrhea	Dysrhythmias
Third-spacing of fluids	Tachycardia
Wound exudates	Ventricular tachycardia
Polyuria	Supraventricular tachycardia
Distributive	Atrial fibrillation
Sepsis	Atrial flutter
SIRS	Bradycardia
Neoplasia	Sinus bradycardia
Pancreatitis	Sick-sinus syndrome
Burns	AV block
Trauma/crush injuries	**Obstructive**
Parvoviral enteritis and other forms of sepsis	Pericarditis (restrictive)
Snakebite/envenomation	Pericardial effusion/tamponade
Immune-mediated hemolytic anemia	Pulmonary thromboembolic disease

The body tries at all times to maintain blood pressure and oxygen delivery. Blood pressure is a function of cardiac output and systemic vascular resistance. Oxygen delivery is a function of cardiac output and arterial oxygen content. Cardiac output is a function of heart rate and stroke volume, where stroke volume is the volume of blood (mL) that the left ventricle ejects in one heartbeat. Stroke volume, in turn, is affected by cardiac preload, cardiac afterload, and myocardial contractility (**105**):

$$Q = \text{Heart Rate} \times \text{Stroke Volume}$$

During states of hypovolemia, the baroreceptors in the carotid body and aortic arch sense a decrease in wall stretch. Wall stretch normally sends a positive feedback to the vagal center in the brain, and causes constant vagal tone to suppress heart rate. When wall stretch is diminished due to a lack of circulating intravascular volume, tonic inhibition of the vagal center is decreased and results in a reflex increase in heart rate. Additionally, by Starling's Law of the Heart, the force of contraction is directly proportional to the effective stretch of the ventricle just before the onset of systole. Thus, the end-diastolic filling volume, which is a function of intravascular fluid volume and return of blood to the heart, is diminished in states of absolute or relative hypovolemia, and will lead to decreased strength of contraction. In an attempt to conserve circulating blood volume to the core tissues, vascular beds will constrict, and can lead to increased cardiac afterload, or the force against which the heart needs to contract. Finally, as the heart beats faster and harder in an attempt to maintain cardiac output, blood pressure, and tissue perfusion during hypovolemia, the heart muscle itself may become fatigued, and lead to depressed myocardial contractility.

Factors that influence blood pressure include cardiac output, as described above, and systemic vascular resistance. Systemic vascular resistance increases when circulating catecholamines released in shock preferentially constrict vascular beds in an attempt to maintain vital perfusion to the heart and brain. Other vascular beds constrict, and oxygen delivery to those tissues diminishes. During states of health, oxygen delivery to tissues meets or exceeds the tissue oxygen demand or needs. In cases of decompensatory shock, however, tissue oxygen extraction becomes dependent on oxygen supply, and thus on oxygen delivery. This is known as supply-dependent oxygen consumption. When oxygen needs or demand exceed supply, tissue oxygen debt, and anaerobic metabolism ensue.

When an animal presents in a state of hypovolemic shock, one must consider where the location of the fluid deficit is. Did the animal actively bleed from a large open wound

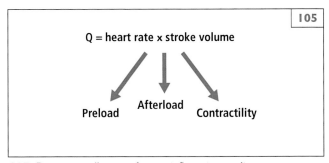

105 Diagram to illustrate factors influencing cardiac output.

or into a body cavity? Conversely, has the animal had such severe vomiting and dehydration that both the interstitial pool and the intravascular pool have become depleted? Normally the interstitial fluid pool will move to the vascular space, and help to maintain serum osmolarity and intravascular fluid volume in the face of an intravascular fluid deficit. The hypothalamus senses an increase in serum osmolality and releases arginine vasopressin (ADH). ADH results in water reabsorption from the kidneys, and helps restore intravascular circulating volume. The actions of ADH are limited, particularly in the face of continued fluid loss. As clinicians, we must intervene to aid in the restoration of intravascular volume in order to improve oxygen delivery.

When an animal has lost less than 25% of circulating blood volume it can still compensate, and usually maintains normal to increased heart rate, normothermia, and normotension. This stage of shock is known as 'compensatory shock' (*Table 44*). As intravascular volume depletion continues, and circulating fluid volume decreases by more than 30%, the body continues to respond in an effort to maintain cardiac output and tissue perfusion. The heart rate will be increased, body temperature will be normal to decreased, and the blood pressure will be normal to decreased. The renin–angiotensin–aldosterone axis will become activated and retain sodium and water. The release of catecholamines such as epinephrine and norepinephrine will cause peripheral vasoconstriction in an attempt to maintain core organ perfusion and oxygen delivery. This stage of shock is known as 'early decompensatory shock' (*Table 44*). Unless interventions are made to restore intravascular fluid volume, the heart will become fatigued; heart rate will then slow and can have dysrhythmias, cardiac output will decrease, blood pressure will continue to decrease, and tissue perfusion will be impaired. The body can compensate only to some degree, and if hypovolemic shock is allowed to continue without replacing intravascular fluid volume, eventually the tachycardic heart muscle will become fatigued and develop a myocardial acidosis. Without the compensatory tachycardia to maintain blood pressure, the patient will become hypotensive and have

decreased tissue perfusion and impaired oxygen delivery. This stage is known as 'late or terminal decompensatory shock' (*Table 44*). Tissue oxygen debt will lead to impaired enzymatic functions and can lead to cell death. Cellular death or dysfunction of any organ system can lead to increased patient morbidity, and if left untreated, can lead to impaired

Table 44
Parameters of shock

Compensatory
  15–30% loss of circulating blood volume
  Hyperemic mucous membranes
  Tachycardia
  Vasoconstriction
  Rapid CRT
  Normal to increased mean arterial pressure

Early decompensatory
  30–40% loss of circulating volume
  Pale mucous membranes
  Tachycardia
  Prolonged CRT
  Normal to decreased mean arterial pressure

Late decompensatory/terminal
  >40% loss of circulating volume
  Pale to gray mucous membranes
  Normal to decreased heart rate
  Prolonged CRT
  Decreased mean arterial pressure
  Poor pulse quality
  Hypothermia

CRT: capillary refill time

function of multiple organs, or multiple organ dysfunction syndrome (MODS).[4]

Treatment of hypovolemic shock involves rapid assessment of the patient's needs, and intravenous or intraosseous administration of some type of fluid or combination of fluids, to restore intravascular circulating volume. Intravenous and intraosseous catheter placement, crystalloid fluids, colloid fluids, blood products, and, if available, hemoglobin-based oxygen carriers have been discussed in other chapters in this text. The physical examination and patient monitoring are extremely important to help determine the degree or extent of shock, whether the patient has an interstitial versus intravascular fluid volume deficit, and can also help to locate the potential cause or source of fluid loss. Too frequently and incorrectly, clinicians use the terms dehydration and hypovolemia interchangeably. Hypovolemia refers to a decrease in intravascular circulating fluid volume. Physical examination abnormalities that are associated with decreased intravascular

fluid volume include pale mucous membranes, delayed capillary refill time, tachycardia or bradycardia, cool peripheral extremities, and hypothermia (*Table 45*).[4] Clinical signs and physical examination abnormalities associated with dehydration are more subjective in nature, and are used as a general gauge to assess interstitial and intracellular dehydration (*Table 46*). Severe dehydration from conditions such as vomiting, diarrhea, unregulated diabetes mellitus, and renal failure can all lead to hypovolemia when the interstitial fluid pool is depleted, and can no longer move into the intravascular fluid pool to restore circulating volume.

More aggressive monitoring can also lend some insight into the extent of poor perfusion, as well as response to therapy. Many animals will be hypotensive. Remember that poor perfusion is equivalent physiologically to impaired oxygen delivery. With tissue oxygen debt, metabolism shifts from aerobic pathways to anaerobic pathways, with lactate produced as a byproduct. Blood pressure, urine output,

---

Table 45
Comparison of parameters of dehydration versus hypovolemia

Dehydration
   Increased skin turgor
   Sunken eyes
   Mucous membrane dryness
Hypovolemia
   Tachycardia
   Prolonged CRT
   Hypotension
   Cool extremities
   Decreased urine output

Table 46
Estimates of dehydration

<5%	History of fluid loss, no abnormalities on physical examination
5%	Dry oral mucous membranes, mild skin tenting
7%	Increased skin turgor, dry oral mucous membranes, mild tachycardia, normal pulses
10%	Increased skin turgor, dry oral mucous membranes, tachycardia, decreased pulse pressure
12%	Markedly increased skin turgor, dry mucous membranes, sunken eyes/dry cornea, alteration of consciousness

and serial lactate monitoring (www.lactate.com) should be considered before and during treatment for hypovolemic shock. Although some studies have demonstrated decreased survival if lactate concentrations are higher than 6.0 mmol/L (54 mg/dL),[5] newer studies have documented that it is better to measure trends in serial lactate concentrations.[6] If an animal's serial lactate is decreasing in response to a particular therapy, therapy should be continued. If lactate concentration is increasing in response to therapy, the prognosis becomes more guarded[6-8] and therapy must become more aggressive or have other changes to help improve perfusion.

When an animal presents in hypovolemic shock, one must consider the location of the fluid deficit, the presence of electrolyte abnormalities, and whether dehydration is a component of a fluid deficit, or if the deficit is associated with the intravascular space alone. If an animal is demonstrating any clinical signs associated with hypovolemic shock (cool peripheral extremities, pale mucous membranes, delayed/prolonged capillary refill time, hypothermia), one of the main differential diagnoses to consider is that cardiogenic shock can cause the same clinical abnormalities. Once cardiac disease has been ruled out, the administration of intravenous or introsseous crystalloid or crystalloid with a colloid is the best method of restoring intravascular fluid volume. Remember that peripheral vasoconstriction is one of the compensatory mechanisms that occurs to maintain circulating central volume. Therefore, administration of subcutaneous fluids is not an efficient means of restoring intravascular volume because of poor and delayed absorption from the subcutaneous space. 'Shock' volumes of intravenous fluids have been recommended for the treatment of hypovolemic shock. Recommended doses are 90 mL/kg in dogs, and 44 mL/kg in cats.[3,9,10] However, the administration of such a large volume of crystalloids can be time consuming, and also dilute out coagulation factors, platelets, and blood cells. Additionally, approximately 75–80% of the crystalloid volume infused will leave the vascular space within 1 hour of administration.[11] Instead of administering a full 'shock volume' of

fluids immediately, it is preferred to administer one-quarter as quickly as possible, then reassess the perfusion parameters. What is the heart rate doing? Is it still elevated, or is it reducing to normal? What is the blood pressure doing? Is it normalizing, or is the patient still hypotensive? Is the animal producing urine? If its kidneys are normal, it will not produce urine until the intravascular fluid volume and renal perfusion have been adequately restored. Is the mucous membrane color returning to normal, or is it still pale, gray, with delayed capillary refill?

If the animal is responding, then one can consider moving to maintenance fluid rates and performing diagnostics to assess and treat the primary cause of the problem. If the animal is not responding, or if the perfusion parameters have not normalized, then an additional one-quarter shock bolus of crystalloid fluids can be administered, or administration of a colloid can be considered. Care must be exercised when administering large volumes of fluids to any patient with hypovolemic shock secondary to hemorrhage, particularly those with signs of closed cavity trauma. Excessive crystalloid fluids can leak out into the interstitial spaces of the lungs and the brain when pulmonary contusions and head trauma are present. Rapidly restoring blood volume and blood pressure to supraphysiologic levels can potentially cause clots that have formed to start bleeding again, and cause worsening of hemorrhage. For these reasons, careful titration of small volumes of crystalloid fluids in combination with colloid solutions, or colloid solutions alone, can be administered as 'small volume resuscitation'.

Small volume resuscitation refers to the administration of small volumes of fluids to restore blood pressure to a mean arterial pressure of 60 mmHg, and preferably, a systolic pressure of approximately 100 mmHg and diastolic pressure of 40 mmHg. Remember that the coronary arteries are perfused during diastole, and require a diastolic pressure of 40 mmHg or more for perfusion. The administration of incremental boluses (5 mL/kg) of synthetic colloids can be used for such a practice. The colloid infused, being large molecular weight particles, will remain in circulation for a much longer period than a crystalloid (see Chapter 4). As such, smaller volumes will need to be administered to restore blood pressure, because the fluid infused will remain attracted around the core structure of the colloid molecule, and be retained within the vascular space. This fluid retention will help maintain blood pressure in the absence of ongoing fluid loss. Synthetic colloids such as hydroxyethyl starch, dextran-70, pentastarch, and hemoglobin-based oxygen carriers (if available) can be administered as an intravenous or intraosseous bolus, and then titrated carefully based on constant reassessment of perfusion parameters.[3] Again, if the perfusion parameters are improving, then further colloid boluses may be unnecessary. Care must be exercised, though, when administering colloids, as hydroxyethyl starch solutions have been shown to bind with von Willebrand factor, and reduce clotting when volumes greater than 40 mL/kg have been administered.[12] This is likely not to be of significant consequence clinically unless the animal is affected by, or a carrier of, von Willebrand's disease.

Hypertonic saline (23.4%) can be diluted with a synthetic colloid at a ratio of 1 part hypertonic saline to 2.5 parts colloid (hydroxyethyl starch, for example), and will create a 7.5% hypertonic saline solution.[9] Hypertonic saline in combination with a synthetic colloid such as hydroxyethyl starch (5–10 mL/kg of the combination in dogs, 2 mL/kg of the combination in cats; total dose in either species should not exceed 1 mL/kg/min as a bolus)[1] can also be used to treat hypovolemic shock initially, provided that the patient is not clinically dehydrated as well.[12] Remember that dehydration refers to interstitial and intracellular fluid deficit. Hypertonic saline acts to increase serum sodium concentration. The body senses the higher serum sodium concentration and lower water concentration relative to that of the interstitium. Water will move by osmosis down its concentration gradient to dilute serum sodium, and move into the intravascular space. By combining the hypertonic saline with a colloid, the fluid that moves into the intravascular space will be retained around the core structure of the colloid, and remain in the intravascular space temporarily, for about 20–30 minutes. Because the fluid has been scavenged from the interstitial and intracellular spaces, the bolus must be followed by the administration of a crystalloid fluid as well, to replenish interstitial and intracellular as well as intravascular fluid pools. Potential complications of hypertonic saline administration include rapid respiratory rate, hypotension, and bradycardia in addition to hypernatremia.[1,13]

CARDIOGENIC SHOCK

Cardiogenic shock is associated with impaired cellular oxygen delivery secondary to defects in cardiac function.[14] This can be associated with various cardiomyopathies, in which myocardial function is impaired, or due to atrial or ventricular dysrhythmias. Cardiogenic shock can also be a secondary adverse sequela of organ failure from other forms of shock, such as septic shock or the systemic inflammatory response syndrome (SIRS), in which circulating inflammatory cytokines can directly impair myocardial function.

The clinical signs, and clinical stages of cardiogenic shock are similar to that observed with hypovolemic shock, and many patients with cardiogenic shock present to the clinician with decompensation and some degree of pulmonary edema (**106, 107**). In addition to cool peripheral extremities, pale mucous membranes, delayed capillary refill time, hypotension and poor pulse quality, and decreased urine output, the patient may have peripheral cyanosis and pulmonary crackles on thoracic auscultation. In left-sided ventricular failure, pulmonary capillary wedge pressure increases and causes extravasation of fluid from the pulmonary vascular beds into the pulmonary interstitium and alveoli. Oxygen cannot diffuse into the pulmonary capillaries to bind with hemoglobin. In addition to poor cardiac output and inadequate delivery of available oxygen to the peripheral tissues, oxygen content of the blood

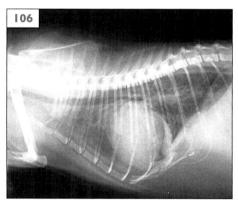

106 Lateral thoracic radiograph of a cat with congestive heart failure secondary to hypertrophic cardiomyopathy and biatrial enlargement. Note the enlarged cardiac silhouette, and the alveolar lung pattern dorsal and caudal to the heart.

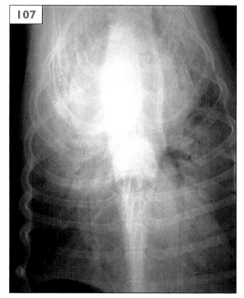

107 Ventrodorsal thoracic radiograph of a dog with congestive heart failure secondary to dilative cardiomyopathy. The globoid cardiac silhouette is difficult to appreciate as it is largely obscured by severe alveolar lung pattern due to pulmonary edema.

will be diminished due to impaired oxygen uptake by the lungs. Cellular extraction of oxygen at the tissues can greatly exceed supply, and large quantities of desaturated hemoglobin (>5 g/dL [50 g/L]) in the peripheral tissues will be observed clinically as cyanosis (**108**).

The treatment of cardiogenic shock differs greatly from that of hypovolemic shock, in that the administration of large volumes of crystalloid or even small volumes of colloid fluids can potentially worsen pulmonary edema. Instead, therapy is first directed at improving oxygen uptake by the lungs. Supplemental oxygen should be administered in the least stressful manner possible (**109**). Second, diuretics such as furosemide (4 mg/kg IV or IM) should be administered to reduce vascular preload and

remove fluid from the lungs. Mild sedation with 0.025 mg/kg IV morphine may be administered to dilate splanchnic vessels and allow a place for fluid to move, as well as to mildly reduce anxiety and the work of breathing. The provision of intravenous fluids is titrated for administration of other inotropic drugs, and to restore interstitial and intracellular fluid deficits caused by the administration of diuretics, once pulmonary edema has resolved. Pimobendan (0.25–0.6 mg/kg PO bid) can be used as a balanced arteriovenodilator and positive inotrope in cases of myxomatous degeneration of the mitral valve, as well as dilative cardiomyopathy in dogs.

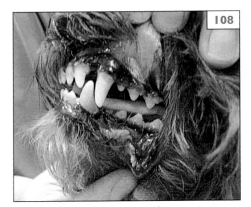

108 Cyanosis of the gums and tongue in a patient with congestive heart failure and pulmonary edema secondary to mitral regurgitation.

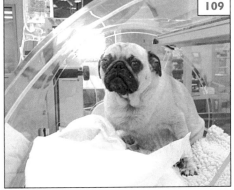

109 Pug in an incubator into which supplemental oxygen is administered. Oxygen flow rates of 50–150 mL/kg/min are recommended. This patient had pulmonary hypertension. Placement of a nasal or nasopharyngeal oxygen tube would be too stressful in any patient with significant respiratory distress.

In addition to the administration of diuretic drugs and oxygen to patients with congestive heart failure, positive inotropic drugs such as dopamine, dobutamine, and ephedrine (*Table 47*) may also be utilized to improve myocardial contractility, particularly in cases of dilative cardiomyopathy (**110**) or poor contractility (**111**) secondary to end-stage left ventricular failure for a variety of causes, including mitral valve disease/regurgitation. Higher doses of positive inotropic drugs, particularly dopamine, may also affect heart rate. Elevated heart rate will not only increase myocardial oxygen demands, but may impair diastolic filling time and coronary artery perfusion during diastole. For this reason, heart rate must be carefully monitored in addition to blood pressure during the infusion of any drug. Sodium nitroprusside is a balanced arteriovenodilator to help dilate vessels and reduce pulmonary capillary wedge pressure and cardiac afterload in the congestive heart failure patient. Because of its

Table 47
Inotropic and vasopressor drugs to improve myocardial contractility and blood pressure

Drug	Use	Dose
Dopamine	Renal perfusion (low-dose)	1–5 λg/kg/min
	Positive inotrope (intermediate)	5–7 λg/kg/min
	Vasopressor (high-dose)	10 λg/kg/min
Dobutamine	Positive inotrope	2–15 λg/kg/min
Norepinephrine		0.5–2 λg/kg/min
Epinephrine		0.1–1 λg/kg/min
Ephedrine		0.1–0.25 mg/kg IV
Phenylephrine		1–3 λg/kg/min

potent vasodilatory effects, sodium nitroprusside must be carefully titrated based on clinical response to therapy and blood pressure. If mean arterial pressure drops to less than 60 mmHg or diastolic pressure to less than 40 mmHg, the dose must be reduced or the drug discontinued. Vasopressor therapy should be considered as a last resort to restore blood pressure in the patient with congestive heart failure. The use of epinephrine, norepinephrine, and vasopressin can potentially increase blood pressure by causing vasoconstriction, increased cardiac preload, and impaired perfusion to tissues. Thus, nonpreferred tissue perfusion may be diminished at the expense of increasing core organ perfusion, as evidenced by improved blood pressure. Additionally, the use of epinephrine, for example, can increase myocardial oxygen demand, and may contribute to myocardial oxygen debt and acidosis.

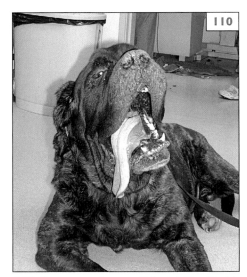

110 Sherman, an 8-year-old English Mastiff with dilative cardiomyopathy. This patient also had atrial fibrillation at the time of presentation, with a ventricular rate of 280 bpm.

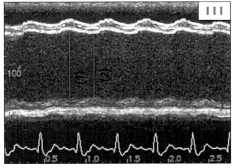

111 M-mode from an echocardiogram of a patient with dilative cardiomyopathy showing left ventricular chamber size during systole (2) and diastole (1). Note that the percentage change is minimal, as contractility is so diminished.

DISTRIBUTIVE SHOCK

Distributive shock is a term used for any condition associated with inappropriately dilated vascular beds. This commonly is secondary to states in which massive inflammation is present, or SIRS. Criteria for SIRS in cats and dogs have been defined (*Table 48*).[15] Septic shock is a SIRS condition specifically related to systemic inflammation in the presence of bacteremia. Bacterial endotoxin, or lipopolysaccharide from Gram-negative bacteria, is a potent stimulator of neutrophils, macrophages, and platelets. Stimulation of the immune cells and platelets further causes the release of inflammatory mediators and vasoactive substances such as platelet-activating factor, interleukins-1, -6, -8, and -10, and tumor necrosis factor.[15] These key players are only a small part of the inflammatory cascade which results in vasodilation, vascular endothelial damage, and myocardial depression, and if left untreated can ultimately lead to impaired microvascular circulation, DIC, MODS, and patient mortality.

Clinical signs of distributive shock differ from those of other forms of shock (hypovolemic, cardiogenic, or obstructive) in that in the early stages of distributive shock, dogs will have very hyperemic mucous membranes (**112**) with tachycardia, rapid capillary refill time, fever/pyrexia, and tachypnea.[15] The clinical signs of distributive or septic shock differ in cats, in that there is hypothermia, bradycardia, and hypotension. Mucous membrane color in cats is often pale, with prolonged capillary refill time.[15,16] Despite the difference in clinical signs, the astute clinician may recognize that distributive shock may be present, depending on the patient's signalment and history. This potentially can be difficult in cats, as cardiogenic and hypovolemic shock often can manifest very similar clinical signs to distributive shock.

Treatment of SIRS and/or septic shock involves first removing the underlying cause. Removal of the inciting cause may involve removal or repair of injured or necrotic tissue, administration of antimicrobial drugs, or inactivation of toxins, in the event of snakebite, for example. Unfortunately, even if the inciting cause is alleviated, the inactivation of the inflammatory response is often delayed, sometimes by days, as tissue heals. One analogy is of sending troops (namely neutrophils, platelets and macrophages) into battle, and having the enemy defeated. The troops' communication lines are patchy, at best, and they cannot hear when they are being recalled, so they keep fighting. Therefore, other treatment is largely supportive in nature until the effects of the inflammatory cascade are eventually suppressed.

Intravenous crystalloid fluids must be used to maintain metabolic fluid requirements and replenish ongoing losses. Large volumes of crystalloids, however, can potentially leak out of the intravascular space into the interstitial space due to disruption in the vascular endothelial membrane. Interstitial edema will further impair tissue oxygen delivery. For this reason, therapy with a balanced crystalloid fluid in combination with a colloid (20–30 mL/kg/day IV CRI) is recommended to help maintain the crystalloid fluid infused in the vascular space. Additionally, depending on the patient's underlying disease and needs, natural colloid support in the form of concentrated albumin, FFP, and/or whole blood or pRBCs may be required to replenish and maintain colloid oncotic pressure (albumin), clotting factors (FFP and whole blood), and antithrombin (FFP and whole blood).

Positive inotropic drugs, such as dobutamine, dopamine, and ephedrine (*Table 47*) may also be required to improve myocardial contractility.[8] Norepinephrine is the pressor of choice to constrict inappropriately dilated vascular beds; however, epinephrine and vasopressin also may be considered. The treatment of SIRS and septic shock is challenging, particularly when there is evidence of end-organ damage distant to the site of inciting cause, and without extremely aggressive therapy, can ultimately lead to the patient's demise.

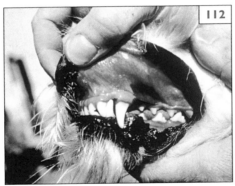

112 Hyperemic mucous membranes in the dog. (Courtesy of Manson Publishing/The Veterinary Press: M. Schaer, *Clinical Medicine of the Dog and Cat*, 2010.)

Table 48
Criteria for systemic inflammatory response syndrome in dogs and cats

If two or more of the following criteria are met in dogs or cats, systemic inflammatory response syndrome (SIRS) is considered to be present. An important note is that the criteria must be taken in the context of the patient's clinical status and recent activity

Criteria	Finding
Respiratory rate	>20 breaths/minute or a $PaCO_2$ <32 mmHg
Temperature	Elevated >103.5°F (39.7°C) or decreased <100°F (37.8°C)
White blood cell count	Elevated >12,000/λL or decreased <1000/λL OR >10% band neutrophils
Heart rate	Tachycardic >160 beats per minute (canine) >250 beats per minute (feline)*

*Note that in some cats with various causes of systemic inflammation, the heart rate may be decreased and bradycardic.

OBSTRUCTIVE SHOCK

Obstructive shock is a shock state secondary to impaired delivery of blood to the right heart or impaired perfusion through the lungs to the left heart.[8] Without delivery of blood to the right heart, and ultimately delivery of blood to the left heart, blood cannot be oxygenated then delivered to the periphery. Conditions associated with obstructive shock include gastric dilatation and volvulus (**113**), in which the large rotated stomach compresses the caudal vena cava and obstructs inflow to the right atrium/ventricle. Heartbase or atrial masses that cause pericardial effusion or pericardial tamponade also commonly obstruct inflow to the right heart. Severe heartworm disease (**114**) can obstruct flow through the pulmonary arteries into the lungs and left heart, and cause caval syndrome. Finally, pulmonary thromboemboli can obstruct inflow into the left heart from the lungs, and aortic tumors or thrombi can obstruct outflow of blood from the left heart. All of the conditions ultimately result in impaired cellular oxygen delivery.

Clinical signs of obstructive shock are similar to those of hypovolemic shock, with pale mucous membranes, delayed or prolonged capillary refill time, tachycardia in compensated shock, bradycardia in decompensated shock, hypotension, and later, hypothermia. The clinical signs should alert the clinician to start therapy at the same time as determining the underlying cause of obstructive shock.

The treatment for obstructive shock largely depends on elimination of the underlying disorder. In the cases of pericardial tamponade or gastric dilatation volvulus, pericardiocentesis or trocarization of the distended stomach can result in improved blood flow to the right heart and improved cardiac output. Surgical removal of heartworms from the pulmonary arteries may be necessary in addition to other adulticide therapies to allow inflow of blood from the right heart to the lungs in cases of severe caval syndrome. In the case of pulmonary thromboemboli, determination of the underlying cause of hypercoagulability is necessary in addition to considering therapies both to dissolve the clots (tissue plasminogen activator, for example) and to prevent further

clots (aspirin, warfarin, heparin, and/or clopidogrel). In the case of aortic tumors or thrombi, surgical intervention may also be necessary, depending on the size and location of the mass or thrombus, in addition to therapies as stated above to dissolve clots and prevent further clot formation. The simplest condition that can cause obstructive shock, unfortunately, is gastric dilatation volvulus, which also has a large component of distributive shock associated with the release of inflammatory cytokines and oxygen-derived free radical species once perfusion to the stomach is restored.

Fluid therapy in obstructive shock is tailored according to the patient's underlying condition and needs. Until pericardial tamponade is resolved, administration of large volumes of intravenous fluids is not likely to be successful in restoring perfusion, because little of the fluid infused will get to the right heart. This also holds true with veno-occlusive disease in caval syndrome, pulmonary thromboembolism, aortic thromboembolism, and aortic tumors. In cases of gastric dilatation-volvulus, however, intravenous crystalloids and colloids, or hypertonic saline with colloids may be administered in the same manner as for hypovolemic shock, titrating the fluid volume administered with restoration of the patient's perfusion parameters.

In any shock state, the use of fluids in combination with treatment of the underlying disease process is mandatory. Additionally, careful monitoring of these patients is required on a moment-to-moment basis until they are stabilized, and frequently thereafter, to ensure that they remain stabilized.

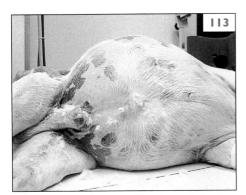

113 Bulldog with gastric dilatation volvulus in lateral recumbency. Note how distended the abdomen appears.

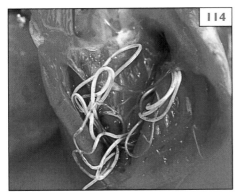

114 Adult heartworms in the ventricle at postmortem. (Courtesy of Manson Publishing/The Veterinary Press: M. Schaer, *Clinical Medicine of the Dog and Cat*, 2010.)

CARE AND 'RULE OF TWENTY'

Dr. Rebecca Kirby published the 'Rule of Twenty'[17] which is a list of 20 very important things to consider when treating any critically ill animal, including those with hemorrhage and/or hypovolemic shock (*Table 49*). The Rule of Twenty can be used on an acute emergency or on a daily basis as a check-list to help maintain an understanding of the intricacies of multi-organ interaction.

Table 49
Original Kirby's 'Rule of Twenty'

1. Fluid balance
2. Blood pressure
3. Heart rate/rhythm and contractility
4. Albumin
5. Colloid oncotic pressure
6. Oxygenation and ventilation
7. Glucose
8. Coagulation
9. Acid–base and electrolyte status
10. Mentation
11. Red blood cell/hemoglobin concentration
12. Renal function
13. White blood cell, immune function, antibiotic dose and selection
14. Gastrointestinal integrity, motility, and function
15. Drug dose and selection
16. Nutrition
17. Analgesia and pain control
18. Nursing care, patient mobility
19. Wound and bandage care
20. Tender loving care

Additional parameters and guidelines are discussed in the text as additional monitoring, for example lactate, has become available.

1 Fluid balance

In animals with the various forms of shock, fluid balance is very important. One must consider the location of the fluid deficit, as well as any ongoing losses that may be present. First, treatment should consist of refilling the vascular space by intravenous or intraosseous administration of crystalloid or colloid fluids, or both. Second, acid–base and electrolyte status may have serious derangements, and the type and components of the fluid chosen should be considered to alleviate abnormalities, and correct interstitial and intracellular dehydration. Once an animal is adequately rehydrated (intracellular and interstitial pools) and volume replenished (intravascular fluid volume restoration), 'ins and outs' can be calculated, taking into consideration the volume of fluid taken in the form of intravenous/intraosseous fluids or oral intake. Fluid eliminated in the form of urine, vomit, and feces can be measured or weighed, using the conversion that 1 mL of fluid weighs approximately 1 g. Additionally, insensible losses in the form of sweat and respiratory secretions should be estimated at 20–30 mL/kg/day. If the fluid intake does not equal fluid loss, either the patient's fluid deficit has not been restored, the kidneys are not functioning correctly, or the animal is third-spacing fluid into the interstitial, peritoneal, retroperitoneal, or pleural space(s). Careful attention should be used when treating distributive shock, as third-spacing of fluids into body cavities or the subcutaneous space may occur due to loss of vascular endothelial integrity. Combination therapy with crystalloids and colloids should be considered, to help maintain fluid in the intravascular space.

2 Blood pressure

Blood pressure is one of the monitoring tools that allows clinicians to make an assessment of presumed perfusion. Blood pressure can be measured directly with an arterial catheter connected to a blood pressure transducer, or can be measured indirectly with a Doppler or an oscillometric monitor. Although normo- or hypertension is not a specific indicator of tissue perfusion, hypotension or trends toward hypotension are important in making decisions when to intervene. As fluid loss becomes severe, blood pressure can drop precipitously. With intravenous fluid replacement, blood pressure should normalize. Ideally, systolic pressures of at least 100 mmHg, diastolic pressures of at least 40 mmHg, and mean arterial pressures of at least 60 mmHg are ideal. If fluid replacement alone does not improve blood pressure, positive inotropic drugs to increase myocardial contractility and vasopressors to cause vasoconstriction can be administered.

3 Heart rate/rhythm, pulse quality, and contractility

During hypovolemic, distributive, and hemorrhagic shock, heart rate initially increases during the compensatory and early decompensatory phases to maintain cardiac output in the face of decreased circulating intravascular fluid volume and decreased cardiac output. As myocardial oxygen demands become elevated, myocardial ischemia can result in local and global acidosis and cardiac dysrhythmias. Vasodilation or vasoconstriction and decreased blood pressure can result in poor pulse quality. Additionally, myocardial contractility can be impaired due to myocardial ischemia, acidosis, and the presence of inflammatory cytokines. Careful monitoring of ECG, blood pressure and pulse quality is an indirect way of assessing cardiac output in the absence of a pulmonary artery catheter. Antiarrhythmic drugs may also be required to control atrial or ventricular dysrhythmias.

4, 5 Albumin and colloid oncotic pressure

Albumin is one of the most important proteins in the body, and is the major contributor to colloid oncotic pressure (COP), or the water-holding pressure in a fluid cavity. Crystalloid fluids do not contain albumin or any source of colloid. During hemorrhage, protein can be lost along with RBCs and fluid, and lead to hypoalbuminemia. Administration of crystalloid fluids alone can dilute albumin, and can contribute to decreased oncotic pressure and extravasation of fluid from the intravascular into the interstitial space, and worsen tissue edema and impaired tissue oxygen delivery. A goal should be to raise serum albumin to at least 2.0 g/dL (20 g/L) with some sort of albumin or (less effectively) with plasma therapy, then use other colloids to help maintain oncotic pressure. Ideally, measurement of COP with a colloid osmometer can be used to gauge therapy.

6 Oxygenation and ventilation

Oxygenation and ventilation can be impaired by pulmonary fluid overload, pulmonary hemorrhage, or pulmonary contusions. During traumatically induced hemorrhagic shock, the potential for other injuries that can impair oxygen delivery to the tissues, including pneumothorax and pulmonary contusions, can also occur. Direct monitoring of arterial blood gases to assess arterial oxygenation, ventilation with CO_2, and calculation of arterial to alveolar oxygen tension gradients (A–a gradient) or P_aO_2/F_iO_2 ratios can help assess the degree of diffusion impairment and decreased ability to oxygenate. In the absence of being able to perform an arterial blood gas, indirect monitoring of hemoglobin saturated with oxygen (S_pO_2) can be performed with pulse oximetry. In animals with hemorrhagic or hypovolemic shock, peripheral vasoconstriction, or hypotension, cool peripheral extremities can lead to artifactual abnormalities in the pulse oximetry readings. If the heart rate that is obtained on the pulse oximeter does not match the patient's actual heart rate, as a rule the S_pO_2 value is likely to be inaccurate. Oxygen supplementation with a face mask, oxygen hood, oxygen cage, or nasal/nasopharyngeal oxygen can be used at a flow rate of 50–150 mL/kg/minute.

7 Glucose

Many animals that have hemorrhagic shock evoke a stress response and the release of catecholamines can cause a stress-induced hyperglycemia. In other instances, severe vomiting and diarrhea, for example as a result of sepsis, can cause increased glucose utilization and hypoglycemia. Glucose should be monitored at least twice a day, or more frequently as warranted by the animal's primary condition and potential need for glucose supplementation. In critically ill human patients, tight glucose regulation with insulin therapy is used to help reduce patient morbidity. Although this concept is novel for veterinary patients, until research is conducted that can prove a decrease in patient morbidity and/or mortality, very tight regulation of glucose control and prevention of hyperglycemia is probably not warranted. Treatment of hypoglycemia, however, is necessary if the patient's blood glucose drops near or below 60 mg/dL (3.33 mmol/L).

8 Coagulation

Depending on the cause of hypovolemia and/or hemorrhagic shock, coagulation can be impaired due to impaired platelet function, thrombocytopenia, or lack of active vitamin K-dependent coagulation factors. A platelet count can be measured directly, or can be measured indirectly by a simple blood smear, and counting the number of platelets per high-power field. Multiplying the number of platelets per high-power field on a peripheral blood smear by 10,000–15,000 will give an estimate of platelet number. When a platelet count drops to less than 50,000/μL, spontaneous bleeding can occur. Other tests of coagulation include an APTT to test the intrinsic clotting cascade, and a PT to test the extrinsic clotting cascade. Factor VII is the factor with the shortest half-life, and can cause the PT to become prolonged before we see any changes in the ACT or APTT. If there is a suspicion of exposure to a vitamin K antagonist rodenticide, and/or a significantly prolonged PT, then replenishment of vitamin K-dependent coagulation factors in the form of cryoprecipitate or FFP and vitamin K may be necessary. Infusion of large volumes of crystalloid fluids, or even massive transfusion[8] in hemorrhaging patients can dilute coagulation factors and platelets and exacerbate a coagulopathic state. In an animal with hemorrhage due to severe trauma or neoplasia, DIC can exist. Although an animal's platelet count may be still within a normal reference range, a trend toward a decreasing platelet count can signal impending DIC.

9 Acid–base, electrolyte, and lactate status

During hemorrhage and hypovolemic shock, decreased tissue perfusion can lead to lactic and metabolic acidosis. Venous pH, electrolytes, and lactate (115) are simple and useful monitoring tools to help assess end-organ perfusion and function. Serial determinations allow the clinician to evaluate the success or lack of success of treatment. While initial lactate concentrations may be extremely elevated, the more important value to obtain and recognize is the lowering of serum lactate in response to therapy as a predictor of patient morbidity and mortality.[6]

115 Lactate monitor.

10 Mentation

When an animal loses more than 30% of its circulating blood volume or has severe dehydration and possible electrolyte abnormalities, mentation changes that range from mental dullness, tremors (hypoglycemia, hypocalcemia), obtundation, coma, or seizures can result. It is sometimes difficult to assess an animal's neurologic function until intravascular fluid volume has been restored, and any electrolyte or hypoglycemia corrected.

11 Red blood cell/hemoglobin concentration

RBC and hemoglobin concentration can be significantly decreased during states of hemorrhagic or hypovolemic shock. However, initially, splenic contraction can raise the PCV by anywhere from 5% to 15%, even in the face of ongoing blood loss. With severe fluid loss in excess of solute, such as that observed with a free water deficit, intravascular fluid loss can be excessive, but severe hemoconcentration with very elevated hematocrits can be observed, as seen in animals with hemorrhagic gastroenteritis. In either case, oxygen delivery can be diminished, and intravascular fluid volume must be restored. If RBC loss is so significant that the patient is clinical for anemia after intravascular volume has been replenished, pRBCs, whole blood transfusion, or administration of a hemoglobin-based oxygen carrier (if available) should be considered.

12 Renal function

Whenever there is excessive blood loss, hypovolemia, and subsequent hypotension, any state that causes impaired oxygen delivery can result in hypoperfusion and impaired renal function. Initially, prerenal azotemia can be observed on blood tests due to poor renal perfusion secondary to hypovolemia. Once intravascular fluid volume has been restored and blood pressure has been normalized, the patient must be carefully monitored. One of the indirect measures of global perfusion is whether the animal is producing urine. Even if the patient is producing urine, observation of glucosuria or renal tubular casts can be an indicator of renal damage, and should be closely monitored. Urine output can be calculated after collection in a closed collection system attached to a urinary catheter (116), or can be estimated by weighing the patient's bedding. Ideally, following correction of intravascular volume status and interstitial fluid deficits, a patient's urine output should be at least 1–2 mL/kg/hour. For patient cleanliness, a urinary catheter is preferred for collection of urine. Provided that the catheter is placed and maintained correctly, the presence of a urinary catheter alone does not necessarily increase the risk of a bacterial urinary tract infection when used short-term.[8]

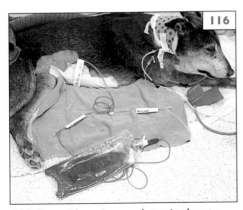

116 Dog with a urinary catheter in place to measure ins and outs while undergoing peritoneal dialysis for leptospirosis. Note the edema on the ventral mandibular region due to interstitial fluid overload.

13 White blood cell, immune system function, antibiotic dose and selection

Any stressor can cause suppression of immune function. Additonally, critically ill animals often have a number of catheters (intravenous, intraosseous, thoracic drainage, urinary, sometimes abdominal drainage or tracheostomy tubes) that penetrate the body's normal defensive barriers to infection. Body fluids in the form of wound exudates, vomit, diarrhea, and blood can also contaminate overlying bandages and wick infection into the patient from the surrounding hospital environment, creating a nosocomial or catheter-induced infection.[18] Depending on the cause of the shock, and whether there are any underlying problems, antibiotics may be indicated. When necessary, the choice should ideally be based on bacterial culture and susceptibility testing.

14 Gastrointestinal integrity, motility and function

The GI tract is the stress organ in dogs, and can also be dysfunctional in cats that have had any cause of hypotension. Mesenteric blood flow can be greatly diminished as the body compensates in an attempt to maintain perfusion to preferred organs such as the heart and brain. Bacterial translocation can result and can cause sepsis, distributive shock, and increased patient morbidity and mortality. Additionally, in the presence of vomiting, diarrhea, or impaired neurologic function, inability to provide enteral nutrition can lead to enterocyte atrophy and bacterial translocation. Antiemetics, gastroprotectant drugs, and provision of enteral nutrition to whatever portion of the GI tract is functional are advised.

15 Drug dose, selection, and metabolism

The administration of numerous drugs is very common in small animal critical care units. Too frequently, however, drugs will interfere with the metabolism or action of one another, and can either reduce the effects of some drugs, or increase the risk of toxicity of other drugs. For this reason, each drug, its dose, its mechanism of action, and its metabolism should be considered on a daily basis to prevent adverse interactions.

16 Nutrition

Nutritional support of the critically ill patient is of paramount importance, as the body needs building blocks from which to heal. Additionally, lack of enteral nutrition can quickly lead to enterocyte atrophy and the risk of bacterial translocation, sepsis, and increased patient morbidity and mortality. The REE should be provided as either enteral or parenteral nutrition, or some combination of the two.

17 Analgesia and pain control

Pain can worsen patient outcome, elevate metabolism, contribute to immunosuppression, and impair wound healing. Even in the presence of hypotension, careful use of opioid drugs such as fentanyl, hydromorphone, or morphine can be beneficial and safe when treating pain in the hypotensive or hypovolemic animal.

18 Nursing care and patient mobilization

Nursing care is perhaps the most important aspect of treatment of any critical patient, even above and beyond any medical intervention, except perhaps fluids. Dependent edema, disuse atrophy, and pulmonary atelectasis can occur if an animal is recumbent. Therefore, frequent changing from side to side, propping the patient on soft bedding to prevent decubital ulcers, and passive range of motion exercises, are just a few of the important aspects of taking care of the critical patient.

19 Wound and bandage care

Strikethrough or moisture on bandages will allow the movement of bacteria and debris from the animal's surrounding environment to any wounds or catheters, and can increase the risk of nosocomial infection. Soiled bandages must be changed immediately, to prevent infection. Any type of catheter bandage, even when not obviously soiled, should be removed to evaluate the site of catheter entry into the body on a daily basis, to make sure that there is no discharge or erythema that can signify catheter- or tube-related infection.

20 Tender loving care

Tender loving care is one of the most important aspects of veterinary critical care. Like humans who have been hospitalized out of their home environment, animal patients too can become depressed, which impairs healing. Nursing care, time outdoors, and visits from family can reduce the stress associated with the hospital environment and subjectively improve the patient's demeanor and outcome.

With careful monitoring, diligence, and the guidelines listed above, animals with hemorrhagic, hypovolemic, distributive, and obstructive shock may have a potentially better outcome, depending on their primary disease and response to therapy.

Case examples for fluid therapy

- **Case 1: Gunther**

- **Case 2: Casey**

- **Case 3: Zeke**

- **Case 4: Buster**

- **Case 5: Lolita**

- **Case 6: Lucky**

- **Case 7: Mango**

- **Case 8: Jake**

- **Case 9: Rocket**

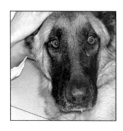 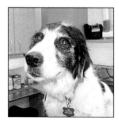 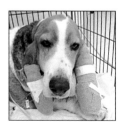 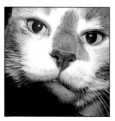

CASE 1: GUNTHER

Gunther, a 10-year-old, 86 lb (39 kg) neutered male German shepherd (**117**), presents with a 1-week history of waxing and waning lethargy and inappetance. His owner reports that today, the dog's abdomen appears to be more distended. He has not eaten today. There has been no vomiting or diarrhea. The owner does not know of any potential exposure to toxins or chemicals. The dog is currently on no medications, is up-to-date on vaccinations, and has had no prior medical problems.

At the time of presentation, his mucous membranes are very pale pink with a prolonged (2.5 seconds) capillary refill time (CRT). His heart sounds slightly muffled, but there are no obvious murmurs or dysrhythmias. His heart rate seems high at 170 beats per minute. The femoral pulses are synchronous and slightly decreased in character. The lungs are clear on thoracic auscultation, and there is no evidence of respiratory difficulty. The abdomen is distended, and there is possibly a ballotable fluid wave. The neurologic and orthopedic and dermatologic systems appear normal at this time.

I. WHAT ARE GUNTHER'S PROBLEMS?
- Waxing and waning lethargy
- Distended abdomen
- Inappetance
- Possible abdominal effusion
- Slightly muffled cardiac sounds

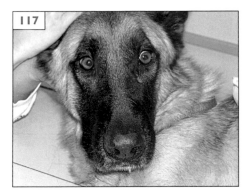

117 Gunther, a 10-year-old neutered male German Shepherd that presents with a 1-week history of waxing and waning lethargy and inappetence.

- Tachycardia
- Decreased pulse quality
- Prolonged CRT

II. WHAT IS GUNTHER'S CARDIOVASCULAR STATUS?
Gunther is showing signs of decompensatory shock, with tachycardia, muffled heart sounds, prolonged CRT, and decreased pulse quality.

III. WHAT IS THE LIST OF DIFFERENTIAL DIAGNOSES?
Differential diagnoses include: neoplasia (hepatic, adrenal, renal, splenic), perforated bowel and peritonitis, cardiac disease (heart failure, pericardial tamponade), pancreatitis, and hepatic failure.

IV. HOW SHOULD GUNTHER BE STABILIZED BEFORE DIAGNOSTIC TESTS?
A peripheral cephalic intravenous catheter is placed, and a one-quarter shock (860 mL) bolus of Normosol-R is administered. To calculate the bolus: a zero is added to a dog's body weight in pounds (i.e. multiply by 10), and that is approximately the 0.25 (90 mL/kg) bolus of a crystalloid to administer during hypovolemic shock. After the one-quarter shock bolus has been administered, heart rate, CRT, mucous membrane color, and blood pressure are reassessed.

His blood pressure is essentially the same, although his heart rate has started to decrease and his mucous membrane color and CRT have improved. A second one-quarter shock bolus of a crystalloid is administered.

V. WHAT IS THE DIAGNOSTIC PLAN?
Initial diagnostic plan includes taking a blood pressure, electrocardiogram (ECG), complete blood count, serum biochemistry panel, urinalysis, thoracic radiographs, and abdominal radiographs, and serum lactate.

Results of diagnostic tests:
- Evaluation of thoracic radiographs shows no abnormalities.
- Complete blood count: 18,580 WBC/μL with 78% neutrophils, 12% lymphocytes, 8% monocytes, and 2% eosinophils; platelet count is 123,000/μL; the hematocrit (Hct) is 32%.

- Chemistry panel is normal except for hyperglycemia glucose 197 mg/dL (10.9 mmol/L), and hypoproteinemia with a total protein 3.8 g/dL (38 g/L).
- Evaluation of the abdominal radiographs show a large soft tissue density in the mid-abdomen, and a decrease in abdominal detail (**118**).
- Reading of the blood pressure showed hypotension with a systolic measurement of 98 mmHg and diastolic measurement of 48 mmHg.

VI. WHAT OTHER PROBLEMS SHOULD BE ADDED TO GUNTHER'S PROBLEM LIST?

- Abdominal mass
- Poor abdominal detail
- Mild thrombocytopenia
- Hyperglycemia
- Hypoproteinemia
- Mild anemia
- Hypotension

VII. WHAT IS THE DIAGNOSIS?

Gunther has a mid-abdominal mass with poor detail, and is showing clinical signs of hypovolemic or hemorrhagic shock.

VIII. WHAT OTHER TESTS COULD BE CONSIDERED?

A blood type is useful, as Gunther maybe has a hemoabdomen based on the loss of abdominal detail, clinical signs referable to hypovolemic/hemorrhagic shock, and the presence of a large mid-abdominal mass effect on radiography.

An abdominocentesis could be performed: nonclotting hemorrhagic fluid is present, which confirms suspicions of hemoabdomen.

IX. WHAT SHOULD BE CONSIDERED NEXT?

Ideally, an abdominal ultrasound and cardiac ultrasound should be performed to rule out the presence of metastases, and to locate the organ from which the mass arises. However, if no ultrasound machine is available, and there are concerns that Gunther may continue to hemorrhage through the night, he should be taken to surgery.

At the time of surgery, a large cavitated splenic mass, with no obvious metastases is found (**119**). A routine splenectomy is performed, and a hematocrit repeated intra-operatively. At this time, Gunther's Hct has dropped to 22%, and he is hypotensive under anesthesia (76 mmHg systolic and 34 mmHg diastolic).

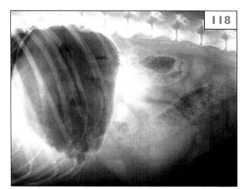

118 Lateral abdominal radiograph showing a soft tissue mass effect in the mid-abdomen.

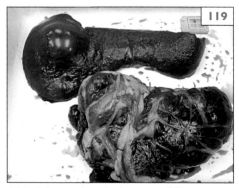

119 Spleen with multiple masses following removal at the time of surgery.

XI. WHAT IS NOW OF CONCERN?

The degree of hypotension and anemia is concerning. Although some of the apparent anemia might be explained from intraoperative crystalloid fluids and hemodilution, anemia with hypotension is dangerous as both can lead to decreased oxygen delivery to the tissues. While the blood typing is being performed, a colloid bolus (5 mL/kg IV) can be administered in an attempt to raise Gunther's blood pressure. A blood transfusion is to be given.

XII. WHAT TYPE OF BLOOD PRODUCT SHOULD BE ADMINISTERED?

Initially Gunther's total protein was low, so fresh frozen plasma (FFP) or frozen plasma may be beneficial to raise the total protein slightly, but he also needs RBCs, so he is given type-specific whole blood. His hematocrit has dropped to 22%, and ideally should be raised to 30% (an 8 percentage point increase from his current Hct). For every 1 mL/lb of whole blood, the Hct will be raised by 1 percentage point. Gunther is 86 pounds, and the Hct should be raised by 8 percentage points, therefore $(8 \times 86) = 688$ mL of whole blood should be transfused. In the clinical situation it is likely that incremental units of whole blood will be administered to be nearly equal to, or slightly more than, the desired calculated volume. If blood is not available, a hemoglobin-based oxygen carrier could also be administered for oxygen-carrying capacity, and as a colloid to augment intravascular fluid volume and blood pressure.

Post-operatively, Gunther does well on maintenance crystalloid fluids, analgesia, and restricted activity until his abdominal incision heals.

CASE 2: CASEY

Casey, a 35 kg (77 lb), 5-year-old neutered male Australian Shepherd/Border Collie mixed breed dog (**120**), presents on emergency referral from another veterinary hospital for possible ethylene glycol intoxication. Casey has been vomiting and having diarrhea for the past 3 days after ingesting 1 lb (0.45 kg) of raisins. The owner reports that there have been raisins visible in the dog's diarrheic feces. Casey has a history of having a sensitive stomach in the past, but no other medical problems. His owner does not know of any chemical or garbage exposure. He is not on any medications except for monthly heartworm prevention.

At the referring veterinary hospital, Casey was initially given subcutaneous fluids and metoclopramide. Blood and urine were obtained for evaluation by an outside laboratory. He was discharged to his owner with instructions to administer a bland diet and to contact them if his vomiting did not resolve. This morning, the blood results were returned, and showed renal azotemia with a BUN 99 mg/dL, creatinine 4.2 mg/dL

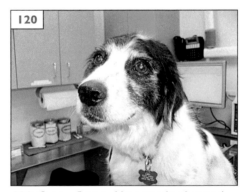

120 Casey, a 5-year-old neutered male mixed breed dog that presents after ingesting 1 lb (0.45 kg) of raisins. He developed vomiting and inappetence, then progressed to anuric renal failure.

(370 μmol/L), his urine specific gravity was 1.018 with glucosuria and amorphous debris, but no white or red blood cells and no bacteria. Urine ketones were negative.

At the time of presentation, Casey is lethargic, and has dry mucous membranes and a normal CRT. His heart rate is 68 beats per minute, and there is a normal sinus rhythm with strong synchronous femoral pulses. He has serous nasal discharge, and slightly edematous conjunctiva. He has halitosis, and vomitus staining around his mouth. Thoracic auscultation reveals normal rhythm and no murmurs. His lungs sound mildly moist with slight crackles. He has pain in his perirenal area on abdominal palpation, and the urinary bladder is small. Rectal examination was normal.

I. WHAT ARE CASEY'S PROBLEMS?
- Vomiting
- Diarrhea
- Overhydration
- Azotemia with low urine specific gravity
- Halitosis
- Serous nasal discharge
- Conjunctival edema
- Relative bradycardia
- Dry mucous membranes
- Harsh lung sounds
- Perirenal pain

II. WHAT IS THE WORKING DIAGNOSIS?
Casey appears clinically overhydrated, yet also has fluid losses in the form of vomiting and diarrhea. Normally, in the face of fluid loss, the kidneys should compensate and retain fluid in an attempt to maintain circulating blood volume. He has a relatively slow heart rate, which could be associated with a number of diseases, including hypoadrenocorticism, hyperkalemia from other causes, including renal failure and uroabdomen, or late decompensatory shock. Although not very sensitive for assessing a patient's actual blood pressure, the presence of very strong pulses makes decompensatory shock less likely. One of the major concerns is primary or secondary renal failure.

III. WHAT SHOULD BE THE INITIAL DIAGNOSTIC PLAN?
Initial diagnostic plans should include an ECG and blood pressure, abdominal radiographs to rule out a foreign body or gastrointestinal obstruction, urethral calculi, or decreased abdominal detail from abdominal effusion. Since the original bloodwork was obtained approximately 24 hours ago, ideally a repeat of the complete blood count, serum biochemical analyses, and urinalysis should be performed, to compare with the bloodwork obtained previously. Thoracic radiographs should be considered because of the moist lung sounds. Whenever renal values are elevated, bacterial infections such as pyelonephritis and leptospirosis should also be considered.

IV. THE ECG IS OBTAINED (121). WHAT DOES IT INDICATE?
This ECG strip represents atrial standstill. Although lone atrial standstill can occur in some breeds of dogs, such as the English Springer Spaniel, the absence of p waves in combination with widened QRS complexes makes hyperkalemia a real concern.

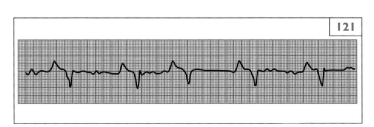

121 ECG tracing from patient with hyperkalemia and acute renal failure. This ECG is characteristic of atrial standstill.

V. BEFORE PERFORMING ANY ADDITIONAL DIAGNOSTICS, WHAT SHOULD BE DONE?

Atrial standstill in a patient with suspected oliguric or anuric renal failure can rapidly become life-threatening if left untreated. Treatment to protect the heart from the toxic effects of hyperkalemia includes the administration of calcium gluconate or calcium chloride IV. Alternatively, potassium can be driven intracellularly with the administration of sodium bicarbonate or IV regular insulin with dextrose. A slow bolus of calcium gluconate was administered over 10 minutes.

VI. WHAT TEST SHOULD NEXT BE PERFORMED?

An oscillometric blood pressure is taken, and shows that Casey is hypertensive, with pressures of 203 mmHg systolic and 120 mmHg diastolic.

The results of the bloodwork have been completed and reveal that Casey's azotemia appears to have worsened. The BUN is 128 mg/dL, and the creatinine is 7.6 mg/dL (672 μmol/L). Casey is also hypercalcemic (total calcium 13 mmol/L [52 mg/dL]) and hyperphosphatemic (>16 mmol/L [50 mg/dL]). The serum potassium is 9.6 mmol/L. Cystocentesis is attempted to provide a urine sample, but is unsuccessful as the urinary bladder is very small. A urinary catheter is placed, and 3 mL of urine obtained. On gross examination the urine appears very light yellow and clear. The specific gravity is 1.006. The sediment examination shows amorphous debris, but no crystals or casts.

VII. ARE THERE ANY ADDITIONAL PROBLEMS TO ADD TO CASEY'S LIST?

- Hypertension
- Atrial standstill
- Hyposthenuria
- Worsened azotemia
- Hypercalcemia
- Hyperphosphatemia
- Small urinary bladder with little urine

VIII. WHAT ARE THE CONCERNS?

In the face of continued vomiting, Casey's azotemia is worsening, and there is little to no urine being produced. He has clinical signs referable to anuric renal failure, with pulmonary crackles, chemosis, and serous nasal discharge. Additionally, his electrolytes are abnormal, with hyperkalemia, hypercalcemia, and hyper-phosphatemia. All of these abnormalities can be attributable to renal failure; however, other diseases such as cholecalciferol rodenticide intoxication and hypoadrenocorticism should also be considered.

IX. COULD THIS BE ETHYLENE GLYCOL INTOXICATION?

Ethylene glycol could cause signs of vomiting, dehydration, azotemia, perirenal pain, hyperkalemia, and hyperphosphatemia. However, with the sedimentation of calcium oxalate crystals in the renal tubules, hypocalcemia, not hypercalcemia would be expected. Additionally, there are no crystals (calcium oxalate monohydrate or calcium oxalate dehydrate, nor hippurate) on the urine sediment examination. Although these findings do not definitively rule out ethylene glycol intoxication, it makes this cause of renal failure less likely.

X. WHAT SHOULD BE THE INITIAL TREATMENT PLAN?

Casey's kidneys should be 'jump started', which is a logistical concern, given the presence of overhydration (chemosis, serous nasal discharge, and pulmonary crackles). Drugs such as furosemide (4 mg/kg IV), mannitol (0.5–1 g/kg IV), dopamine (3–5 μg/kg/min IV CRI), and diltiazem (0.1–0.5 mg/kg IV slowly, then 1–5 mcg/kg/min) have been reported to aid in the production of urine. Some, like diltiazem, also have been used to promote diuresis in patients with renal failure, and have the added benefit of reducing hypertension.

XI. HOW MUCH FLUID SHOULD CASEY RECEIVE? ARE THERE ANY CONCERNS?

Casey is already showing signs of anuria and volume overload. Additional fluids to a volume overloaded patient can worsen pulmonary edema. However, the kidneys need fluid to make urine, and some fluid therapy along with drugs to promote diuresis is in order. If only insensible losses (0.3 mL/kg/hr) are taken into consideration, then (35 kg × 0.3) = 10 mL/hr should be administered.

In acute renal failure, calcium is thought to promote perpetuation of renal damage. Calcium channel blocking drugs such as diltiazem have been recommended to treat hypertension in oliguric or anuric renal failure patients. Casey is placed on a diltiazem constant-rate infusion and his blood pressure monitored very carefully, as patients can become very hypotensive. Administration of furosemide (2–4 mg/kg IV, followed by a constant-rate infusion 0.7–1 mg/kg/hr) can also be considered. The use of mannitol in an anuric patient with signs of intravascular volume overload is contraindicated, as the osmotic effects can draw fluid into the intravascular space from the interstitial space and worsen volume overload.

XII. WHAT IS A SUITABLE MONITORING PLAN?

Measurement of central venous pressure (CVP) allows monitoring of trends and whether Casey has the potential to develop worsened pulmonary edema. A jugular catheter is introduced, and the placement checked with a lateral thoracic radiograph (**122**).

The catheter appears to be in the correct position, with the tip sitting just outside the right atrium. An initial CVP is 8 cmH$_2$O. There does not appear to be obvious interstitial to alveolar infiltrates in the lungs that would suggest pulmonary edema. However, the radiographic appearance of pulmonary edema can lag behind the onset of clinical signs of tachypnea, serous nasal discharge, and chemosis. CVP should be monitored carefully, at least once an hour during the initial phase of fluid therapy, and Casey's respiratory rate and demeanor also reassessed. Measuring body weight every few hours compared with baseline is also a good way to assess rehydration and volume status.

The urinary catheter is kept in place and urine output measured. Normal urine output for a hydrated animal is 1–2 mL/kg/hr. If anuria is suspected, and the interstitial and intravascular fluid deficits have been corrected, 'ins and outs' can be measured, i.e. the amount of fluid taken in (in Casey's case, 193 mL/hr) compared with the amount of fluid Casey puts out in the form of urine, vomitus, and insensible losses (20–30 mL/kg/day).

XIII. WHAT FLUID REPLACEMENT IS BEST FOR CASEY?

Casey has hyperkalemia, hypercalcemia, azotemia, and hyperphosphatemia. Ideally, a fluid that does not contain calcium or potassium should be considered, in the form of 0.9% NaCl. Normal (0.9%) saline promotes excretion of both calcium and potassium.

XIV. SHOULD ANYTHING ELSE BE CONSIDERED?

Casey is still in atrial standstill, and although the 0.9% NaCl will dilute some of the potassium and promote excretion, the toxic

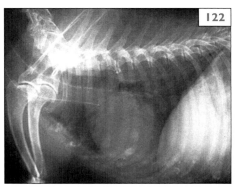

122 Lateral thoracic radiograph of a patient with a jugular catheter whose tip sits just outside the right atrium.

effects of the hyperkalemia can lead to cardiac arrest. Calcium gluconate has already been administered to protect the heart, and intravenous regular insulin combined with dextrose could be given, to drive the potassium intracellularly.

Within 3 hours, Casey's CVP has elevated to 11 cmH$_2$O, but his blood pressure has decreased to 170 mmHg systolic, 80 mmHg diastolic. There appears to be a slow trickle of urine from his urinary catheter into his urine collection bag. CVP above 10 cmH$_2$O greatly increases the risk of impending pulmonary vascular overload. However, as no one value is absolute, the trend in CVP combined with what this animal is doing clinically is perhaps more important. If the CVP rises by more than 5 cmH$_2$O from baseline in a 24 hour period, or if the value is above 10 cmH$_2$O and the animal is becoming more tachypneic with pulmonary crackles, worsening nasal discharge, peripheral edema, and/or chemosis, the clinical picture is more grim.

Casey appears to be improving, and a renal biopsy is recommended. A Tru-cut percutaneous, ultrasound-guided renal biopsy is performed. Histopathologically, the renal tubules are blocked with amorphous debris. There is evidence of mitosis at the glomerular basement membrane, suggesting that the kidneys are improving and attempting to regenerate (**123**).

Many substances can cause insult to the kidneys. Raisins and grapes have been found to be toxic in some animals. The exact toxic dose, and toxic principle are unknown. However, classic clinical signs associated with renal failure from grape or raisin ingestion include vomiting, diarrhea with grape skins or raisins in the feces, and the development of oliguric or anuric renal failure. Renal tubular obstruction appears to be a component of the oliguria or anuria. As the kidneys recover, an overwhelming post-obstructive diuresis can occur, making calculation of fluid ins and outs an absolute necessity.

After 24 hours of intravenous fluids and replenishment of the fluid deficits, 'ins and outs' are calculated, and show that output was 1 mL/kg/day initially, and has increased to 8 mL/kg/day 12 hours later.

XV. WHAT SHOULD BE DONE?

The fluid rate in must match the fluid coming out, so constant monitoring is required to keep up with Casey's enhanced output. Casey should be weighed at least three to four times a day. Rapid changes in body weight are always associated with fluid loss or gain in animals with vomiting, diarrhea, wound exudates, and renal failure.

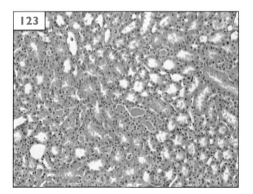

123 Histopathology slide from Casey's kidneys. Histopathologic analysis showed clogging of renal tubules with debris, in addition to regeneration of the renal basement membrane.

CASE 3: ZEKE

Zeke, a 70 lb (32 kg), 4-year-old neutered male Bassett Hound (**124**), presents with an acute onset of collapse. His owners report that he had been normal earlier today, and had access to a fenced-in back yard while they were out of the house. He was found approximately 1 hour ago, collapsed and obtunded in the back yard. His owners report that there were several piles of vomit on the back porch, and brown liquid diarrhea near Zeke. To their knowledge, he had not had any exposure to chemicals, toxins, or garbage. There has been no diet change. Recently in the past 2 months, they had placed Zeke on a diet because of obesity. He has lost a small amount of weight. No other abnormalities were noted until his owners found him.

On physical examination, Zeke is morbidly obese, and obtunded. His mucous membranes are brick red and dry, with a severely prolonged CRT of almost 4 seconds. You find that it is difficult to hear his heart on thoracic auscultation. His temperature, pulse, and respiration are: 97.4ºF (36.3ºC), 120 bpm, and 40 respirations/minute.

I. WHAT ARE ZEKE'S PROBLEMS?
* Obesity
* Obtunded
* Dry mucous membranes: brick red mucous membranes
* Prolonged CRT
* Vomiting
* Diarrhea
* Hypothermia
* Inappropriate bradycardia

II. WHAT IS THE WORKING DIAGNOSIS?
Causes of vomiting and diarrhea are numerous, and include dietary indiscretion, toxin, anaphylactic reaction, inflammatory bowel disease, GI obstruction (including foreign body, intussusception or neoplasia), pancreatitis, bacterial or viral gastroenteritis or secondary to some other infection, mesenteric volvulus, renal or hepatic failure, and metabolic insults such as diabetic ketoacidosis or hypoadrenocorticism.

Zeke is showing signs of neurologic problems with circulatory compromise. The heart sounds are muffled, which can be due to pericardial effusion, pneumothorax, pleural effusion, or hypovolemia. His mucous membranes are brick red, which often is suggestive of septic shock. In the face of dehydration and/or septic shock, one would expect his heart rate to be elevated, unless in the case of end-stage decompensatory shock, where the heart rate can become bradycardic. Inappropriate bradycardia can be associated with a number of conditions, and is significant in this case because Zeke appears to be very hypovolemic. The body's normal response to a decrease in intravascular volume is to compensate with an increase in heart rate in an attempt to maintain cardiac output and blood pressure. Inappropriate bradycardia can be associated with decompensatory shock, increase vagal tone, or electrolyte abnormalities such as hyperkalemia and hypermagnesemia.

His obesity may not be directly associated with his current problems, however, it may impair diagnosis and treatment of his illness.

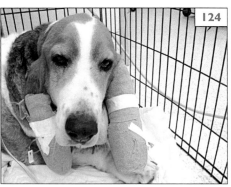

124 Zeke, a 4-year-old neutered male Bassett Hound with an acute onset of collapse.

III. WHAT IS THE INITIAL DIAGNOSTIC PLAN?

The initial diagnostic plan in any patient with severe vomiting, diarrhea, and collapse should include blood pressure, ECG, complete blood count, biochemistry profile, electrolytes, urinalysis, fecal flotation and cytology, thoracic radiographs, abdominal radiographs, and possibly an abdominal ultrasound.

IV. WHAT IS A SUITABLE INITIAL TREATMENT PLAN?

Initial treatment plan in any animal with a history of vomiting, diarrhea, and collapse should include administration of intravenous fluids. Blood samples should ideally be obtained at the time of initial presentation, before the administration of intravenous fluids.

Attempts are made to place peripheral cephalic, lateral saphenous, and medial saphenous catheters, and all are unsuccessful because of patient anatomy, peripheral vasoconstriction, and the severity of obesity.

V. WHAT ALTERNATIVES CAN BE TRIED?

If peripheral vascular access is impossible, a central catheter in the jugular vein can be attempted. Alternatively, a cutdown over an appropriate vessel is another alternative.

Attempts to place a jugular catheter are thwarted, as the degree of obesity prevents catheterization.

VI. IN AN ATTEMPT TO PROVIDE INTRAVENOUS FLUIDS AS SOON AS POSSIBLE, ARE THERE ANY OTHER LOCATIONS IN WHICH A CATHETER CAN BE PLACED?

Intraosseous catheters can be used in patients in whom vascular access is difficult or impossible. Unfortunately, because Zeke is so obese, and because his bones are ossified, it will likely be difficult to place and maintain an intraosseous catheter. Instead, an attempt is made to place an auricular catheter in Zeke's ears. Fortunately it is successful, and two 20-gauge catheters are inserted in the right and left ears, and intravenous crystalloid fluid bolus administration is started.

VII. WHAT FLUID SHOULD BE ADMINISTERED?

In the case of decompensatory shock, it is important first to establish that there is no cardiac disease (in this case, the absence of cardiac sounds makes pericardial effusion a possibility), then administer a balanced crystalloid fluid such as lactated Ringer's, Normosol-R, Plasmalyte-A, or 0.9% sodium chloride. A one-quarter 'shock' bolus of fluid (700 mL in Zeke's case, as he weighs 70 lb) is given, and perfusion parameters of CRT, heart rate, blood pressure, and urine output are reassessed.

The blood panel results are relatively normal except for a hypocholesterolemia (77 mg/dL [2 mmol/L]), hypoglycemia (63 mg/dL [3.5 mmol/L]), hyponatremia (123 mmol/L), hypochloremia (78 mmol/L), and hyperkalemia (7.2 mmol/L).

The ECG rhythm strip shows a normal sinus rhythm despite the presence of hyperkalemia. It is important to note that atrial standstill can be present even with mild hyperkalemia, and the absence of atrial standstill or the presence of a normal sinus rhythm does not rule out the presence of hyperkalemia.

Thoracic radiographs are obtained, and evaluation shows a mild to moderate increase in interstitial to alveolar infiltrates consistent with pneumonia, with a megaesophagus.

VIII. WHAT IS THE LIKELY DIAGNOSIS?

Zeke's signalment and history, being a young Bassett Hound with an acute onset of collapse, vomiting and diarrhea, combined with radiographic appearance of megaesophagus, and bloodwork abnormalities of azotemia, hypocholesterolemia, hypoglycemia, hypo-natremia, hypochloremia, and hyperkalemia are very common in animals with hypo-adrenocorticism, or Addison's disease. None of the aforementioned findings are patho-gnomonic for Addison's, however, and definitive diagnostic testing in the form of an adrenocorticotropic hormone (ACTH) stimulation test must be performed.

One of the interesting and often commonly overlooked 'abnormalities' on the bloodwork of an Addisonian patient is a normal complete blood count. In an animal with severe dehydration, hypovolemia, and collapse, the stress response would result in the demargination of white blood cells (WBCs), and cause a classic stress leukogram with a neutrophilic leukocytosis and lymphopenia. A normal leukogram in a critical patient is an abnormal finding until proven otherwise. The absence of a stress leukogram in an ill patient should increase the index of suspicion for hypoadrenocorticism. In a patient with pneumonia, likely due to aspiration of vomitus, WBCs could potentially infiltrate the diseased lungs, and a leukocytosis may not be present. A neutrophilia should still be present relative to lymphocytes, however.

IX. HOW SHOULD ZEKE BE TREATED?

Treatment of the hypovolemic shock in the form of intravenous crystalloid fluid boluses is of paramount importance. First, the decompensatory shock should be treated with crystalloid fluid boluses (one-quarter shock increments) until the blood pressure has normalized. A colloid such as hetastarch (5 mL/kg increments) can also be administered. If both colloid and crystalloid are unsuccessful in raising blood pressure, positive inotropic drugs or vasopressors may be necessary.

Ideally, administration of 0.9% sodium chloride should be considered to promote potassium excretion. The hypoglycemia can be treated with supplemental dextrose (2.5%) mixed in with the crystalloid fluids. Antiemetic drugs can be administered to treat the vomiting, and broad-spectrum antibiotics and supplemental oxygen can be administered to treat the pneumonia. Careful monitoring of Zeke's glucose and electrolytes should be performed at least twice to three times a day, to avoid continued hypoglycemia or too rapid correction of serum sodium that can lead to central pontine myelinolysis. Definitive treatment of hypoadrenocorticism includes replacement of glucocorticosteroids in the form of prednisone, and replacement of mineralocorticoid activity in the form of fludrocortisone acetate (Florinef) or desoxycorticosterone pivalate (DOCP). Dexamethasone-sodium phosphate (0.5 mg/kg IV) is administered, as it will provide glucocorticoid support and will not interfere with the ACTH stimulation test.

CASE 4: BUSTER

Buster, a 13-year old neutered male domestic shorthaired cat (**125**), presents with a 2-week history of intermittent vomiting, inappetance, and possible weight loss. He is a strictly indoor cat who shares his household with a Pug. There is no possibility of toxin, chemical, garbage, plant, or foreign body ingestion to his owner's knowledge.

At the time of presentation, Buster is in poor body condition, with a relatively unkempt haircoat. His mucous membranes are fairly dry and there is moderate dental calculus and gingivitis. He has increased skin tenting. The muscle mass around his head and dorsal spinous processes are more prominent. On auscultation a grade II– III/VI left parasternal murmur with strong pulse quality and no dysrhythmias is evident. His lungs sound clear. Although he still appears overweight, the kidneys may be slightly small but are not painful on abdominal palpation. His urinary bladder is large, but not tense or painful.

I. WHAT ARE BUSTER'S PROBLEMS?
- Vomiting
- Inappetance
- Muscle wasting
- Dehydration
- Dental calculus and gingivitis
- Murmur
- Possibly small kidneys

II. WHAT TESTS SHOULD BE PERFORMED?
Diagnostic tests would include a complete blood count, biochemistry panel, urinalysis, thoracic radiographs, echocardiogram, and possibly an abdominal ultrasound.

Thoracic radiographs are taken (**126**). There is a classic valentine shape to the heart on the dorsoventral view. An ultrasound appointment with a radiologist is booked in 2 days to have an echocardiogram performed.

A complete blood count revealed a WBC of 14,280 with 82% segmented neutrophils, 13% lymphocytes, and 5% monocytes. Platelet count was normal at 178,000/µL. There was some clumping of platelets at the feathered edge of the blood smear. The hematocrit was 32% with a total protein of 8.2 g/dL (82 g/L). The biochemistry panel revealed significant azotemia

with BUN 125 mg/dL, creatinine 5.6 mg/dL (495 µmol/L), and hypokalemia 3.2 µmol/L. The urinalysis showed a urine specific gravity of 1.018 with some rods and WBCs in the urine.

III. WHAT IS BUSTER'S UPDATED PROBLEM LIST?
- Valentine-shaped heart consistent with hypertrophic cardiomyopathy
- Anemia relative to dehydration
- Azotemia
- Hypokalemia
- Isosthenuria
- Bactiuria
- Pyuria

The degree of anemia initially does not seem severe in the context of the hematocrit alone (32%). However, when the anemia is considered in the presence of clinical signs of dehydration and hyperproteinemia, the anemia is likely significant. A reticulocyte count can be performed to determine whether the anemia is regenerative or nonregenerative.

IV. WHAT FURTHER TESTS SHOULD BE PERFORMED?
Given that there are bacteria and WBCs on the urine sediment examination, a urine culture is in order to determine whether a urinary tract infection or pyelonephritis is contributing to Buster's clinical signs and bloodwork abnormalities. An abdominal ultrasound should also be performed to look at the kidneys and urinary bladder. Ideally, the ultrasound should be performed prior to the administration of intravenous fluids, as dilation of the renal pelves, or pyelectasia, can occur with pyelonephritis and with intravenous fluid therapy.

Some clinicians empirically double or triple the patient's maintenance fluid requirements when treating an animal with chronic renal failure. In many cats with chronic renal failure, empiric calculation of intravenous fluid volume, rather than taking the time to calculate out a fluid deficit, maintenance needs, and ongoing losses, can lead to dehydration in the face of therapy. Intravenous fluid therapy is necessary to replenish interstitial hydration, as well as diurese uremic toxins out of the body that are causing Buster to feel nauseated and vomit. Buster is approximately 7% dehydrated. He weighs 6 kg

(13 lb). To determine the hydration deficit the following formula is used:

$$\begin{aligned}
\text{Deficit (mL)} &= (\text{body weight in kg} \times \% \\
&\quad \text{dehydration}) \times 1000 \\
&= (6 \times 0.07) \times 1000 \\
&= 420 \text{ mL deficit}/24 \text{ hr} \\
&= 17.5 \text{ mL/hr}
\end{aligned}$$

To calculate his maintenance fluid requirements:

$$\begin{aligned}
\text{Maintenance fluids} &= (30 \times \text{body weight in} \\
&\quad \text{kg}) + 70 = \text{mL/day} \\
&= (30 \times 6) + 70 \\
&= 250 \text{ mL/day or} \\
&\quad 10.4 \text{ mL/hr}
\end{aligned}$$

Adding the deficit + maintenance = 17.5 mL/hour + 10.4 mL/hr = 29 mL/hr

V. IS ANYTHING ELSE OF CONCERN?

Buster has a cardiac murmur and signs of biatrial enlargement on the thoracic radiographs. Overzealous administration of intravenous crystalloid or colloid fluid can evoke congestive heart failure with pulmonary edema, pleural effusion, or both in a previously asymptomatic patient. Placement of a jugular or medial saphenous long catheter such that the tip of the catheter sits just outside the right atrium or in the caudal vena cava can be used to measure CVP in cats. Monitoring for trends in change from baseline (no more than 5 cmH_2O increase from baseline within 24 hours) as well as the actual CVP, changes in patient's body weight, and clinical signs of impending pulmonary edema such as tachypnea, increased respiratory effort, pulmonary crackles, serous nasal discharge, or

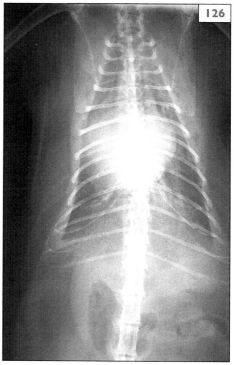

126 Ventrodorsal thoracic radiograph showing classic biatrial enlargement, or a 'valentine-shaped' heart with hypertrophic cardiomyopathy.

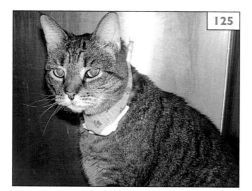

125 Buster, a 13-year-old neutered male domestic shorthaired cat with a history of vomiting, inappetance, and weight loss.

chemosis should all be used together to aid in preventing pulmonary vascular overload.

In Buster's case, however, it is prudent to be a little more cautious, with frequent patient assessment, daily monitoring of renal values, and careful monitoring of body weight and CVP. Usually, renal values will not decrease significantly within the first 48 hours of aggressive fluid therapy. If the renal values are increasing in the face of such therapy, the prognosis worsens. After 48 hours, ideally the renal values will continue to decrease until a plateau is reached. Once a plateau is reached, gradually reducing the patient's intravenous fluids by 25% per day is advised, in order not to reduce fluid support and diuresis too quickly.

In addition to Buster's renal insufficiency and cardiac disease, he has electrolyte imbalance in the form of hypokalemia, which can contribute to muscle weakness. The intravenous fluids should have potassium chloride supplemented, for a dose not to exceed 0.5 mEq/kg/hr.

After 48 hours of crystalloid fluid therapy at a rate of 29 mL/hour, Buster clinically appears more comfortable, and the vomiting has ceased. His body weight has increased by 0.5 kg (1 lb), and his BUN and creatinine have decreased to 56 mg/dL and 3.2 mg/dL (283 μmol/L), respectively. Overall, his CVP has not risen above 5 cmH$_2$O. As Buster has responded well, treatment is continued.

CASE 5: LOLITA

Lolita, a 35 kg (77 lb) 10-month-old spayed female Labrador Retriever (**127**), presents from another veterinary hospital, where she has been hospitalized for the past 3 days. She was spayed 6 days ago, and her owners left her Elizabethan collar off for approximately 1 hour when they left the house. Upon their return, they found Lolita had chewed her midline abdominal incision, and had chewed on a portion of her jejunum. The veterinarian at the other hospital performed emergency surgery on Lolita, and needed to remove approximately 9 inches (23 cm) of damaged jejunum. She had appeared to be doing better and was eating for her owner, until this morning, when she was found to be extremely lethargic with brick red mucous membranes and a prolonged CRT. There was vomitus in her cage, and stained around her muzzle. Her rectal temperature is 104ºF (40ºC). Her heart rate is 160 bpm, and her respiratory rate is 60 per minute. Her abdomen is tense and painful on palpation despite intermittent hydromorphone (0.1 mg/kg IV q6 hr).

I. WHAT ARE LOLITA'S PROBLEMS?
- Recent jejunal resection and anastomosis
- Lethargy
- Vomiting
- Fever
- Tachycardia
- Tachypnea
- Brick red mucous membranes
- Short CRT
- Tense painful abdomen

II. WHAT IS THE LIKELY CLINICAL SITUATION?
Given Lolita's recent surgery 3 days ago, tachycardia, tachypnea, abdominal pain, and brick red mucous membranes with a short CRT and vomiting, there is a strong possibility that Lolita's jejunal incisions have dehisced and she has peritonitis. She has signs of septic shock.

III. WHAT SHOULD BE DONE?
Ideally, an abdominal ultrasound should be performed to evaluate the abdomen for pockets of fluid. A blind abdominocentesis

could be useful: if there is more than 5–7 mL/kg abdominal effusion, there may be a positive tap.

A blind abdominocentesis is performed and fluid obtained (**128**).

IV. WHAT IS THE NEXT STEP?
This fluid is yellow and grossly cloudy, and looks like pus. A cytologic examination of the fluid should be performed.

The fluid is consistent with septic peritonitis, with degenerative neutrophils and intra- and extracellular bacteria.

V. IS SURGERY INDICATED?
Given all of the clinical signs and cytologic examination of the fluid from the abdomen, Lolita requires surgery to re-explore her abdomen.

VI. WHAT ARE THE CONCERNS ABOUT WHICH TREATMENTS TO IMPLEMENT?
Lolita requires intravenous fluids. She has lost fluid into her peritoneal cavity, and also from vomiting and lack of appetite for the past 5 days, until she ate a sesame bagel for her owner yesterday. Intravenous crystalloid fluids to replenish her estimated 7% dehydration deficit are ideal. She also has an intravascular fluid deficit, as evidenced by her prolonged CRT. While it is possible to calculate her interstitial hydration deficit, it is more important, at this time, to treat her intravascular fluid deficit. One-quarter of a 'shock bolus' of crystalloid fluids (Normosol-R, by adding a '0' to her body weight in pounds) is administered, and also a bolus of hydroxyethyl starch (5 mL/kg IV). It is essential to replenish her intravascular fluid deficit before the administration of any negative inotropic, negative chronotropic, and vasodilatory anesthetic drugs for surgery.

Lolita also has a great potential to lose electrolytes and albumin into the peritonitis fluid. She is also at risk for DIC due to the loss of the natural anticoagulant antithrombin into the abdominal fluid, and may become hypoglycemic from sepsis; serum glucose should be monitored at least two to three times per day, and if necessary, additional glucose can be added to the parenteral crystalloid fluids.

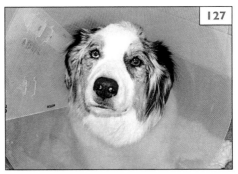

127 Lolita, a 10-month-old spayed female Australian Shepherd with a history of intestinal resection and anastomosis after dehiscence of her spay incision.

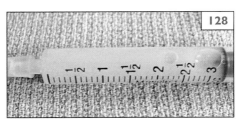

128 Syringe of purulent fluid from Lolita's abdomen, obtained via abdominocentesis.

VII. HOW SHOULD LOLITA'S COLLOID AND PROTEIN SUPPORT BE APPROACHED?
Albumin and colloid oncotic pressure (COP) are important in wound healing. COP can be maintained by using natural and synthetic colloids. FFP only provides a small amount of protein in the form of albumin, some clotting factors, and very small amounts of antithrombin. FFP is often cost prohibitive to replace albumin. Therefore, concentrated human or canine-specific albumin should be administered to replenish serum albumin up to a level of 2.0 g/dL (20 g/L). In the case of septic shock, with the potential for loss of clotting factors in the peritoneal effusion, administration of FFP to replenish clotting factors can be used in combination with albumin concentrates, crystalloid fluids, and a synthetic colloid to help

maintain COP. A synthetic colloid such as hydroxyethyl starch also should be considered to maintain COP by adding 20–30 mL/kg/day IV CRI to the fluid therapy regimen. Because hetastarch and albumin are both colloids that will help retain the fluid administered in the intravascular space, the calculated fluid dose should be reduced by 25–50%. That is, instead of administering 153 mL/hr, 0.75(153) = 115 mL/hr should be given initially, and body weight assessed at least two to three times per day. Lolita's 'ins and outs' can also be monitored by quantitating the amount of fluid in the Jackson–Pratt bulbs ('grenades') and urine output plus an estimate of insensible losses, then determine how much fluid she is receiving in the form of intravenous fluids. In Lolita's case, given that she may not eat immediately, nutrition in the form of a jejunostomy tube or parenteral nutrition with a central catheter should also be considered. One of the best remedies to mediate hypoalbuminemia is to provide amino acids as building blocks for nutritional support. Finally, broad-spectrum antibiotic coverage will be necessary until the results of abdominal cultures are returned.

VIII. IS THERE ANYTHING TO BE CAUTIOUS ABOUT WITH THE ABOVE STRATEGY?
The use of concentrated human albumin is controversial, as all dogs that receive concentrated human albumin can produce anti-albumin antibodies, and have immediate or delayed reactions. Careful observation of Lolita is necessary, to check for the development of clinical signs of vasculitis, urticaria, lames, and joint effusion within days to weeks of receiving concentrated human albumin. Reactions do not occur in all cases, but when they do, they should be treated with anti-inflammatory doses of glucocorticoids, tapering the dose slowly over 3 weeks.

CASE 6: LUCKY

Lucky, a 5-year-old 25 lb (11.3 kg) neutered intact male Cocker Spaniel (**129**), presents on referral for a possible mid-abdominal mass, and anemia. Lucky became lethargic yesterday, and developed a moist cough. His owner took him to another veterinary hospital this morning when she noticed blood-tinged urine. Lucky had abdominal radiographs performed to rule out cystic calculi, and a large soft tissue density was observed in the middle of the abdomen. The other veterinary hospital suspects that there is a splenic mass, and refers for a splenectomy.

At the time of presentation, Lucky is extremely weak with significant respiratory distress. He has scleral hemorrhage, white mucous membranes, and agonal respirations. He is intubated, and an ECG and blood pressure cuff are applied. There is no palpable blood pressure, but an astute technician places a peripheral cephalic intravenous catheter while a preliminary physical examination is being performed.

As well as the scleral hemorrhage, white mucous membranes, and agonal respirations, epistaxis, bradycardia, weak femoral pulses, and bruising in the inguinal region are noted. Lucky urinates, and the urine appears bright red in color.

I. WHAT ARE LUCKY'S PROBLEMS?
- Weakness
- Lethargy
- Cough
- Anemia
- Possible mid-abdominal mass
- Hematuria
- White mucous membranes
- Scleral hemorrhage
- Hypotension
- Agonal respirations
- Bruising
- Epistaxis
- Weak femoral pulses

II. WHAT IS HAPPENING WITH LUCKY?

The presence of acute onset of clinical signs of a coagulopathy in multiple organ systems (scleral hemorrhage, possible hematuria, pale mucous membranes, and possible mid-abdominal mass effect) is very suspicious for a vitamin K antagonist rodenticide intoxication or possibly immune-mediated thrombo-cytopenia.

III. WHAT CAN BE DONE TO CONFIRM A SEVERE COAGULOPATHY?

A full coagulation panel usually consists of a platelet count, prothrombin time (PT), activated partial thromboplastin time (APTT), D-dimers, and fibrin degradation products (FDPs). However, two tests can be performed quickly and efficiently that can evaluate the patient for the two major causes of clinical bleeding, in this case, vitamin K antagonist rodenticide intoxication versus immune-

mediated thrombocytopenia, include an activated clotting time (ACT), and a blood smear to evaluate for the presence of thrombocytopenia.

IV. WHAT ELSE NEEDS TO BE DONE?

Simultaneously with the blood tests being performed, Lucky needs respiratory help, as agonal respirations are nonfunctional and do not sufficiently aerate the lungs. Additionally, Lucky is showing signs of classic hemorrhagic/hypovolemic shock, with pale mucous membranes, very weak pulses, and clinical signs of bleeding. Although he may need RBCs, 250 mL (one-quarter of a 'shock' bolus) of intravenous Normosol-R is administered, to refill the vascular space.

The initial bolus of fluids only slightly improves mucous membrane color and CRT. He is still hypotensive.

V. WHAT CAN BE DONE NEXT?

Lucky needs both intravascular volume and oxygen-carrying capacity. A bolus of type-specific whole blood can be transfused, or, if available, 5 mL/kg of a hemoglobin-based oxygen carrier can be given. Fresh whole blood is given, as it will provide both vitamin K-dependent coagulation proteins as well as RBCs with oxygen-carrying capacity. Whenever there is a patient that is actively hemorrhaging, there is a therapeutic quandary where administration of too little product may not restore blood pressure and perfusion, and too rapid administration of too large a quantity of product can potentially cause dilutional coagulopathies, or can increase the blood pressure and cause clots that have formed to leak off and contribute to active hemorrhage. For this reason, blood pressure monitoring should be used at all times, to resuscitate the patient to a specific blood pressure, ideally 100 mmHg systolic, more than 40 mm Hg diastolic, and a mean arterial pressure of 60 mmHg.

Lucky's platelet estimate is 8–10 per high-power field, and the PT is too high for the analyzer to read.

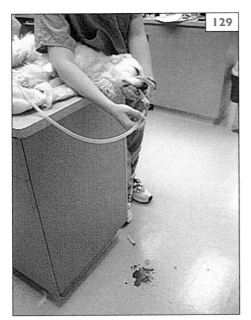

129

129 Lucky, a 5-year-old neutered male Cocker Spaniel, presented with apparent hematuria and significant respiratory distress secondary to pulmonary hemorrhage.

VI. WHAT IS THE LIKELY CLINICAL SITUATION?

A platelet estimate of 8–10 per high-power field is roughly equivalent to 80,000–150,000 platelets/μL. Clinical bleeding does not occur spontaneously until the platelet count falls to 50,000/μL or lower. The PT is a test of the extrinsic clotting cascade, namely, factor VII, the vitamin K-dependent coagulation factor that has the shortest half-life in circulation, and becomes depleted the fastest in cases of vitamin K antagonist rodenticide toxicity. Lucky's owner now asks if Lucky's problems could possibly be related to vitamin K antagonist rodenticide intoxication, because the other dog in the household is currently being treated with vitamin K1 for exposure to the rodenticide!

VII. WHAT TREATMENT SHOULD NOW BE GIVEN?

Treatment for vitamin K antagonist rodenticide toxicity consists of replacing activated vitamin K-dependent coagulation factors (II, VII, IX, X), vitamin K, and intravascular fluid volume. Ideally, the use of FFP is necessary to treat Lucky, at a dose of 10–15 mL/kg. While the plasma is thawing in a tepid water bath, Lucky starts to breathe spontaneously on his own, and his color is improving. His systemic blood pressure has increased to 80 mmHg systolic, and 45 mmHg diastolic. Oxygen supplementation is continued, and 5 mg/kg vitamin K1 administered in multiple subcutaneous sites, with a very small-gauge needle.

VIII. WHAT IS THERE TO DO NEXT?

Lucky still needs the plasma, and although it is ideal to start any transfusion slowly to monitor for signs of reaction, Lucky is in dire need of the coagulation factors, as he is bleeding severely internally, and has experienced respiratory arrest once already. Additional fluid boluses may be helpful in replenishing intravascular volume depletion but will do little to combat the hypocoagulability. The plasma is given as fast as it can be infused, to replenish clotting factors and help stop active bleeding.

IX. WHEN SHOULD THE PROTHROMBIN TIME BE CHECKED?

The PT usually starts to normalize very quickly after the transfusion of FFP is completed. In some cases, depending on how low the hematocrit has fallen, a transfusion of whole blood and/or pRBCs may be necessary. Continued therapy with vitamin K1 (2.5 mg/kg PO bid) for 4–6 weeks is necessary until the vitamin K antagonist rodenticide is fully metabolized and excreted from the body.

As activated vitamin K-dependent coagulation factors, intravascular fluid volume, vitamin K, and supplemental oxygen are administered, Lucky continues to improve dramatically and is soon extubated. Within 2 days, his condition normalizes, and he is discharged to his owner with his long-term vitamin K1 therapy.

CASE 7: MANGO

Mango, a 4-year-old spayed 4 kg (8.8 lb) domestic Shorthaired cat (**130**), presents within 30 minutes of being hit by a car. Her owner reports that she ran under the wheels, seemed to roll under the car, then ran into the neighbor's yard across the street. She initially seemed ambulatory and awake, but has since become more lethargic. She has had no prior health problems, and she is not currently on any medications.

At the time of presentation, Mango has miotic pupils that are sluggishly responsive to light, and is obtunded. A brief physical examination notes that her mucous membrane color is pink with a normal to fast CRT. Her heart and lungs auscult normally, with no murmurs or dysrhythmias, and good lung sounds in all lung fields. There is no sign of orthopnea. Her abdomen is soft and nonpainful, and there are strong synchronous femoral pulses. Within 5 minutes of presentation, Mango throws her head back and has a grand mal seizure.

I. WHAT ARE MANGO'S PROBLEMS?
- Trauma/hit by car
- Miotic pupils with sluggish pupillary light reflex
- Seizure

II. WHAT IS THE WORKING DIAGNOSIS?
The history of trauma, miotic pupils and obtundation that progresses to a seizure should raise the suspicion of increased intracranial pressure and cerebral swelling. As trauma elicits a stress response, catecholamine release can result in increased plasma glucose and hyperglycemia. In cats, the degree of hyperglycemia after head trauma may be adversely associated with clinical outcome. Hypoglycemia can also cause seizures when the blood glucose falls to less than 60 mg/dL (3.33 mmol/L). However, in this case, given the circumstances, hyperglycemia is more commonly expected. A blood glucose is performed to rule out hypoglycemia as a cause of the seizure.

III. WHAT TESTS SHOULD BE DONE?
First, placing a peripheral medial saphenous venous catheter to gain vascular access is extremely important, so that anticonvulsant drugs can be administered. Placing a catheter in the jugular vein is contraindicated, as occluding the vessel to place the catheter can reduce venous outflow from the head, and exacerbate increases in intracranial pressure. Additionally, placing a catheter anywhere in front of the diaphragm can potentially be dangerous to personnel if anticonvulsant drugs need to be administered to an animal that can bite during a seizure episode. A blood pressure and ECG should also be recorded.

Cerebral perfusion pressure (CPP) is a measurement of mean arterial pressure (MAP) minus intracranial pressure (ICP). Perfusion is a result of a pressure differential at different ends of a tube. Cerebral perfusion will decrease as a result of decreased MAP, or increased ICP. Therefore, to maintain cerebral perfusion, one must implement treatment strategies to increase MAP, reduce ICP, or both. Although the brain has a special autoregulatory mechanism to avoid changes in cerebral perfusion in conditions of low MAP or increased ICP, autoregulation does not overcome impaired perfusion in all cases. Because the calvarium or skull is essentially a closed vault, there are very few parameters that can be altered to maintain constant pressure within the skull. These include the brain

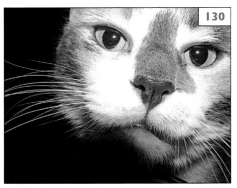

130 Mango, a 4-year-old spayed female domestic Shorthaired cat, presented after being hit by a car.

parenchyma, blood, and cerebrospinal fluid (CSF). As pressure increases, the volume of skull contents must decrease in order to maintain ICP. Since blood flow is autoregulated, and CSF is a constant, rapid changes in ICP can result in herniation of the brainstem through the back of the foramen magnum. Additionally, the body compensates to avoid increases in cerebral blood flow by a reflex decrease in heart rate as ICP rises. When the systemic blood pressure is extremely elevated, heart rate will reflexively decrease due to increased vagal tone, in an attempt to reduce cerebral blood flow and ICP. This is called Cushing's reflex, and is a grave prognostic sign unless emergency measures are implemented.

The ECG shows a sinus bradycardia with a heart rate of 51 beats per minute, and a systolic blood pressure of 230 mmHg is obtained. This is very characteristic of Cushing's reflex. Mango's blood glucose is 280 mg/dL (15.5 mmol/L), consistent with a stress hyperglycemia.

IV. WHAT SHOULD BE DONE NOW?

Diazepam (1.25 mg IV) is administered, and supplemental oxygen is given by mask over Mango's face. Nasal prongs and nasal tubes are contraindicated because of the risk of sneezing and increasing ICP. Administration of a glucocorticosteroid to lower ICP is contraindicated, as there has been no documented benefit of administration of steroids in head trauma patients, and the effect can worsen hyperglycemia and cerebral acidosis. Instead, 3 mL/kg of hypertonic saline is given as a bolus over 15 minutes, as hypertonic saline reduces cerebral edema and draws fluid from the interstitial space into the intravascular space. After the hypertonic saline, 5 mL/kg IV hetastarch is given, then maintenance (8 mL/hr) lactated Ringer's solution. After 10 minutes, Mango's systemic blood pressure starts to decrease, and her heart rate increases to 120 bpm.

V. IS THERE ANYTHING ELSE THAT CAN BE DONE?

Mango seems to be responding to the hypertonic saline. However, mannitol (0.5–1 g/kg) can also be administered as an osmotic diuretic to reduce cerebral edema. After administration of mannitol (0.5 g/kg), Mango's pupil size increases slightly, and she begins to become more responsive. Although she is far from being 'out of the woods', she seems to be improving.

Hypertonic saline is a fluid that should be considered in cases of severe head trauma. Because its effects are short-lived, intravenous colloids need to be administered to have a sustained effect, to prevent the fluid that has been pulled into the intravascular space from the interstitial and intracellular space flowing back into its primary location. Because fluid can be pulled from the intracellular space, continued therapy with an intravenous crystalloid is necessary to replenish intracellular electrolytes and fluid.

The 'Rule of Twenty' monitoring and nursing care is implemented, as Mango's condition is still very critical. Mango is placed on a stiff board, and her head elevated by 20º by placing a towel under the board. With some care, there is a chance that Mango could survive.

CASE 8: JAKE

Jake, a 1-year-old, 22 kg (48 lb) intact male Pembroke Welsh Corgi (**131**), presents approximately 20 minutes after being hit by a car. The vehicle was moving at approximately 40 miles per hour (64 km/h), and his owner said that Jake was struck on the left side. He was thrown into the air, then ran to the neighbor's yard, where he lay down. His owner has noticed some abrasions on his legs, and increased respirations. He did not lose consciousness, and has not urinated or defecated since the accident. To date, he has not had any other medical problems, and is not on any medication.

On physical examination Jake is ambulatory, and tachypneic with a respiratory rate of 60 respirations per minute. His respirations are rapid and shallow. His mucous membrane color is grayish pink, with a CRT of slightly more than 2 seconds. He is tachycardic with a heart rate of 160 beats per minute with strong synchronous pulses. His lungs sound harsh on the left side. His abdomen and limbs palpate normally, with no obvious fractures, and no soft tissue swelling. There are no obvious neurologic deficits.

I. WHAT ARE JAKE'S PROBLEMS?

- History of being hit by a car
- Abrasions
- Tachypnea
- Tachycardia
- Harsh lung sounds
- Gray mucous membranes
- Prolonged CRT

II. WHAT SHOULD BE DONE INITIALLY?

For any patient that has been struck by a moving vehicle there are concerns about the possibility of internal and external injuries, including a pneumothorax, pulmonary contusions, diaphragmatic hernia, internal hemorrhage, ruptured urinary bladder, and avulsed organs. He has the potential to develop myocardial contusions and traumatic myocarditis with cardiac dysrhythmias that can reduce cardiac output and blood pressure. Therefore, ideally blood pressure and ECG should be measured to obtain baseline readings, and he should be monitored for signs of hypotension and cardiac dysrhythmias. Remember the 'ABCs' of trauma and emergency: stablize the airway and breathing, then address circulation. Jake's respiratory and circulatory status must be stabilized prior to performing diagnostic tests.

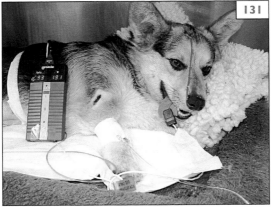

131 Jake a 1-year-old Welsh Corgi that presents after being hit by a car.

In all animals that have been hit by a car, thoracic and abdominal radiographs should be performed after initial stabilization, to rule out a diaphragmatic hernia, pneumothorax, and pulmonary contusions. Baseline bloodwork that consists of a complete blood count and serum biochemical analyses should also be performed at the time of presentation, in the event that if the patient's condition worsens, a baseline sample is available for comparison.

Jake's ECG shows a sinus tachycardia, and his blood pressure is 80 mmHg systolic, and 43 mmHg diastolic. Blood has been obtained, and bloodwork currently is running in the laboratory. His Hct is 48%, and total protein is 6.2 g/dL (62 g/L).

III. WHAT ELSE NEEDS TO BE ADDRESSED?

Jake's hypotension must be treated. Placement of a peripheral cephalic IV catheter is advocated in any traumatized patient on presentation. Even the most 'stable' animals can decompensate very quickly if there is internal hemorrhage.

IV. WHAT SHOULD BE ADMINISTERED TO JAKE?

Ideally, a one-quarter shock dose of intravenous crystalloid fluids should be given initially to improve blood pressure. The full shock bolus is 90 mL/kg; Jake weighs approximately 48 lb, so a one-quarter shock bolus is 480 mL of a balanced crystalloid such as lactated Ringer's. One other thing to consider is that Jake is already showing signs of pulmonary contusions. A pulmonary contusion is essentially a large bruise in the lungs, and can worsen both clinically and radiographically over the next 24–48 hours. Overzealous fluid administration can worsen the edema in the lungs, and contribute to ventilation–perfusion mismatch and hypoxemia.

Instead, a bolus of 5 mL/kg (110 mL) colloid such as hetastarch is given, and his perfusion parameters of heart rate, CRT, mucous membrane color, and blood pressure are reassessed. Hypertonic saline (3 mL/kg) could also be given with the colloid bolus, for a short-lived movement of fluid from the interstitial space into the intravascular space.

V. IS THERE SOMETHING ELSE THAT CAN BE DONE?

Jake is hypoxemic, his oxygen saturation is low, and can be remedied by supplemental oxygen. Supplemental oxygen can be administered by an oxygen cage, flow-by oxygen, oxygen hood, or nasal or nasopharyngeal oxygen. Nasopharyngeal humidified oxygen is given, at a rate of 100 mL/kg/minute. Jake's respiratory rate and effort improve after the onset of supplemental oxygen. In any traumatized patient, and in particular those that display any signs of respiratory distress, administration of supplemental oxygen is one of the first things that should be employed, even as as physical examination occurs.

During this time, Jake's blood pressure has improved to 100 mmHg systolic, and 54 mmHg diastolic after his fluid bolus.

VI. WHAT SHOULD BE OBTAINED NEXT?

Thoracic radiographs should be obtained (**132**). No obvious abnormalities are found on abdominal radiographs.

VII. WHAT IS THE DIAGNOSIS AND WHAT TREATMENT SHOULD BE IMPLEMENTED?

A pneumothorax. Ideally, whenever there is a pneumothorax, the air should be removed with thoracocentesis. Both sides of the thorax should be aspirated, until negative pressure is obtained on both sides. If negative pressure cannot be obtained, of if there is frequent reaccumulation of air that is causing increased respiratory effort and respiratory compromise, a thoracic drainage catheter or thoracostomy tube should be placed.

In Jake's case, pain, anxiety due to increased work of breathing, and the pneumothorax can all potentially be contributing to the hypotension, and although he is hypotensive, analgesia should definitely be administered to control discomfort. A dose of hydromorphone (0.1 mg/kg IV) is administered to control discomfort.

Next, a thoracocentesis is performed by quickly clipping both sides of Jake's chest and inserting a needle into the thorax in the seventh intercostal space, and withdrawing the air from both sides until negative pressure is reached. Although there is improvement in the respiratory rate and effort, Jake still has a restrictive respiratory pattern with pulmonary crackles. His oxygen saturation by pulse oximetry is 86% on room air.

VIII. HOW SHOULD TREATMENT CONTINUE?

Jake's blood pressure is normal at this time. It should be closely monitored. However, overzealous fluid administration can be detrimental and contribute to free lung water. Therefore, administration of maintenance fluids at a rate of (30 mL/day × BW in kg) + 70 mL/day is recommended, with constant reassessment of perfusion parameters in the event of further possible internal hemorrhage. The rest of the treatment consists of supportive care and tincture of time until the bruises in Jake's lung heal and he can be taken off supplemental oxygen.

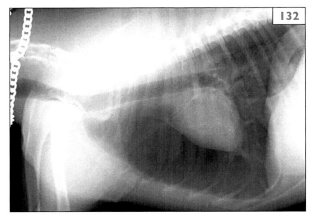

132 Lateral thoracic radiograph demonstrating elevation of the heart from the sternum and retraction of the lung lobes, with pneumothorax, after being hit by a car.

CASE 9: ROCKET

Rocket, a 5 kg (11 lb), 10-week-old Australian Cattle Dog puppy (**133**), presents with a 2-day history of vomiting white froth and bilious fluid, and diarrhea that has now become hemorrhagic. His owner has attempted to feed him water with an eye dropper, but the puppy promptly vomits. Before now, the puppy was active and healthy, and took daily walks to the dog park. His owner states that he has received two vaccinations from the breeder. There is no possibility of having ingested any toxins, chemicals, or garbage, and she has not changed his diet recently. There is no known ingestion of any toys or other foreign objects, and no ingestion of table scraps.

Physical examination reveals that the puppy is severely lethargic, with pale pink-white dry mucous membranes, and a prolonged CRT. His eyes appear sunken in the orbits, with no apparent ocular discharge. There is no nasal discharge, and the lungs sound normal with no apparent respiratory difficulty. The heart auscults normally with no murmurs or dysrhythmias. On palpation the abdomen feels doughy with no palpable masses. However, the intestines feel as if they are fluid-filled. There is blood-tinged diarrhea in the perineal region. The puppy's skin tents and remains in place for more than 1.5 seconds before slowly returning to its normal place.

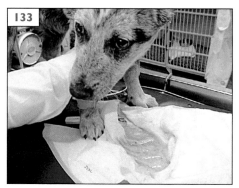

133 Rocket, a 10-week-old Australian Cattle Dog that presented with vomiting and hemorrhagic diarrhea.

I. WHAT ARE ROCKET'S PROBLEMS?
- Vomiting
- Diarrhea (bloody)
- Lethargy
- Pale, dry mucous membranes
- Dehydration
- Hypovolemia
- Prolonged CRT

I. WHAT TESTS SHOULD BE PERFORMED?
GI viruses such as parvovirus and coronavirus, GI parasites, toxins, and foreign bodies and GI obstructions are possible diagnoses. A test for parvovirus and complete blood count, serum electrolyte and glucose are recommended, and the puppy started on intravenous fluids.[1] As the parvovirus fecal antigen ELISA test is running, an intravenous catheter is placed.

II. WHAT TYPE OF CATHETER SHOULD BE PLACED?
Although a peripheral catheter may be easier to place, it is likely to become soiled with vomitus and diarrhea. A jugular catheter is preferable, as it is less likely to become soiled and is relatively easy to place, and is well tolerated, even by puppies. In addition, frequent blood samples will be needed to check serum glucose and electrolytes, and a central catheter will allow this without the need for repeated venipuncture. It is important to note that if placement of the jugular catheter will delay treatment, placement of a peripheral catheter, or an intraosseous catheter, should be considered until a jugular catheter can be placed more easily.

There are a variety of single- and multi-lumen catheters available. A multi-lumen catheter will allow a variety of fluids and blood products such as plasma to be administered, if necessary. In addition, its central location will allow provision of hyperosmolar solutions such as parenteral nutrition in this debilitated puppy.

III. HOW MUCH FLUID (ML/H) SHOULD BE ADMINISTERED?

Given the presence of dry mucous membranes, sunken eyes, extreme skin tenting, tachycardia, and mild hypothermia, the puppy's dehydration deficit is estimated at approximately 10%. Once an animal is sufficiently dehydrated that they develop tachycardia, intravascular hypovolemia has occurred. Maintenance fluid needs, and ongoing losses should also be calculated.

$$5 \text{ kg} \times 0.1 \times 1000 = 500 \text{ mL deficit}$$
$$500 \text{ mL deficit}/24 \text{ h} = 21 \text{ mL/hr}$$

$$\text{Maintenance fluids per day} = (30 \times \text{body weight in kg}) + 70$$
$$= (30 \times 5) + 70 = 220 \text{ mL/day}$$
$$= 220 \text{ mL}/24 \text{ hours} = 9.2 \text{ mL/hr}$$

Ongoing losses:

Remember that 1 mL of vomitus or diarrheic feces weighs approximately 1 g. A reasonable method to assess ongoing losses is to weigh bedding before placing it into the cage, then weighing it as it becomes soiled. The best method of assessing whether the puppy's ongoing losses are being matched is to weigh him frequently, at least three times a day, to make sure that he is not losing weight despite fluid therapy.

IV. WHAT TYPE OF FLUID SHOULD BE ADMINISTERED?

This puppy requires replacement of both intravascular and interstitial fluid deficits. Although he is not currently hypoalbuminemic, he has the potential to lose a great deal of protein through his GI tract until the diarrhea ceases. A balanced replacement crystalloid fluid such as Normosol-R is recommended.

V. SHOULD ANY ADDITIVES BE INCLUDED?

The puppy will likely lose electrolytes in his diarrhea and feces. At this time, his serum potassium is normal, although that could change and so must be carefully monitored. Potassium (20 mEq KCl/L) is added. The puppy's lack of enteral nutrition and frequent vomiting is of concern, and he may become hypoglycemic. Until the puppy's vomiting decreases in frequency, nasogastric feeding is not advised. However, a nasogastric tube can be used to suction the fluid from the stomach, and reduces vomiting by preventing gastric overdistension. Enteral nutrition is always preferred over microenteral nutrition. Microenteral nutrition, by trickle feeding small amounts of amino acid solution or balanced enteral feeding product such as Clinicare, can be beneficial even if the puppy is still vomiting. Small amounts of microenteral nutrition to the enterocytes has been show to improve survival and reduce the length of hospital stay in puppies with parvoviral enteritis.[1]

VI. IS THERE ANYTHING ELSE TO BE CONSIDERED?

Enteral nutrition is preferred over parenteral nutrition, but the puppy is vomiting profusely. Although it is easier to supply dextrose as an additive in crystalloid fluids, small amounts of dextrose (2.5–5%) in intravenous fluids simply supplies enough glucose to maintain serum glucose above 60 mg/dL (3.3 mmol/L). The dextrose does not provide sufficient calories to maintain the puppy's metabolic energy requirements. Therefore, he needs parenteral nutrition.

VII. WHAT IS THE PUPPY'S RESTING ENERGY REQUIREMENT?

Resting energy expenditure (REE) is the same as the metabolic water requirement, as it takes 1 mL of water to metabolize 1 kcal of energy.

$$\text{REE} = (30 \times \text{body weight in kg}) + 70$$
$$= (30 \times 5) + 70 = 220 \text{ kcal/day}$$

Because the puppy is supposed to be growing, it is not improper to consider multiplying this value by 1.2–1.4. However, oversupplementation of calories in the form of carbohydrate may be detrimental as he needs to excrete more carbon dioxide. It is decided to administer the REE on the first day, and consider making changes the next.

VIII. HOW SHOULD THE PARENTERAL NUTRITION BE FORMULATED?

The parenteral nutrition should provide 20% of the calories as dextrose, 80% of the calories as lipid, and 3 g of protein per 100 kcal of energy.

Dextrose: 20% of REE
$= (0.2 \times 220) = 44$ kcal as dextrose, and 50% dextrose is 1.7 kcal/mL
$= 44$ kcal $\times 1$ mL/1.7 kcal $= 26$ mL 50% dextrose

Lipid: 80% REE
$= (0.8 \times 220) = 176$ kcal as lipid, and 20% lipid is 2 kcal/mL
$= 176$ kcal $\times 1$ mL/2 kcal $= 88$ mL 20% lipid

Protein: Provide 3 g per 100 kcal of energy
$= 220/100 \times 3 = 6.6$ g protein, and 8.5% amino acid solution contains 0.085 g protein/mL
$= 6.6$ g protein $\times 1$ mL/0.085 g protein
$= 77$ mL 8.5% amino acid solution

Adding them all together:
26 mL 50% dextrose
88 mL 20% lipid
77 mL 8.5% amino acid $= 191$ mL

191 mL/24 hr $= 7.95$ or ≈ 8 mL/hr parenteral nutrition solution

This can be administered in a designated line, or possibly combined as a total nutrient admixture, incorporating it into the puppy's daily fluid requirements, whichever is easier. Remember that it will still be necessary to add in any ongoing fluid losses. If a multi-lumen catheter is available and multiple pumps, the parenteral nutrition can be provided as a solution by itself. However, if only a single-lumen catheter and a limited supply of fluid pumps are available, then it may be easier to give it as a total nutrient admixture along with the fluids.

IX. IS THERE ANYTHING ELSE TO TAKE INTO CONSIDERATION?

In any puppy with the potential for electrolyte and fluid deficits, hypoglycemia, compromised immune system, and potential for bacterial translocation and sepsis, a 'Rule of Twenty' monitoring plan is necessary to make sure that fluid loss, glucose and energy requirements, and electrolyte abnormalities are all addressed. A first-generation cephalosporin and enrofloxacin, or a cephalosporin plus metronidazole, a second-generation cephalosporin, or a β-lactam such as ampicillin with enrofloxacin are all good choices for the provision of broad-spectrum antibiotics for this puppy. To medicate the vomiting, potent antiemetic drugs such as dolasetron (0.6 mg/kg IV once daily) or maropitant (1 mg/kg SQ, 2 mg/kg PO), along with metoclopramide (1–2 mg/kg/day IV CRI) should also be administered. Although the puppy's serum albumin concentration may be normal in the face of dehydration, it may quickly decrease with loss in diarrheic feces. For this reason, some clinicians would empirically start colloidal support in the form of a hydroxyethyl starch solution (20 mL/kg/day IV CRI) in addition to the parenteral nutrition and crystalloid fluids. Bandage care is of paramount importance, as puppies with parvoviral enteritis can quickly soil catheter bandages, and the fecal material or vomitus can wick through the bandage to the catheter site and cause contamination and infection.

References

CHAPTER 1

1 Wellman ML, DiBartola SP, Kohn CW (2006). Applied physiology of body fluids in dogs and cats. In: DiBartola SP (ed). *Fluid, Electrolyte, and Acid–Base Disorders in Small Animal Practice*, 3rd edn. Saunders Elsevier, St Louis, pp. 3–26.

2 Mazzaferro EM, Rudloff E, Kirby R (2002). Role of albumin replacement in the critically ill veterinary patient. *J Vet Emerg Crit Care* 12(2):113–124.

3 Kern MR (1997). Osmolarity, hyperosmolarity. In: Tilley LP, Smith FWK Jr (eds). *The 5-Minute Veterinary Consult*, 2nd edn. Lippincott, Williams & Wilkins, Philadelphia, pp. 310–311.

4 Silverstein DC (2009). Daily intravenous fluid therapy. In: *Small Animal Critical Care Medicine*. Saunders-Elsevier, St. Louis, ch 64, pp. 271–275.

5 de Morais HA, Biondo AW (2006). Disorders of chloride: hyperchloremia and hypochloremia. In: DiBartola SP (ed). *Fluid, Electrolyte, and Acid–Base Disorders in Small Animal Practice*, 3rd edn. Saunders Elsevier, St Louis, pp. 80–90.

6 Wingfield WE (2002). Fluid and electrolyte therapy. In: Wingfield WE, Raffe MR (eds). *The Veterinary ICU Book*, Teton Newmedia, Jackson Hole, ch 13, p. 170.

7 Walton RE, Wingfield WE, Ogilvie GK, Fettman MJ, Matteson VL (1996). Energy expenditure in 104 postoperative and traumatically injured dogs with indirect calorimetry. *J Vet Emerg Crit Care* 6(2):71–79

CHAPTER 2

1 Davis H (2009). Central venous catheterization. In: Silverstein DC, Hopper K (eds). *Small Animal Critical Care Medicine*. Saunders-Elsevier, St. Louis, ch 63.

2 Davis H (2009). Peripheral venous catheterization. In: Silverstein DC, Hopper K (eds). *Small Animal Critical Care Medicine*. Saunders-Elsevier, St. Louis, ch 61.

3 Giunti M, Otto CM (2009). Intraoosseous catheterization. In: Silverstein DC, Hopper K (eds). *Small Animal Critical Care Medicine*. Saunders-Elsevier, St. Louis, ch 62.

4 Otto CM, Kaufman GM, Crowe DT (1989). Intraosseous infusion of fluids and therapeutics. *Comp Cont Educ Pract Vet* 11(4):421–424.

5 Hackett TB, Mazzaferro EM (2006). *Veterinary Emergency and Critical Care Procedures*, Blackwell Scientific, London.

6 Mazzaferro EM (2009). Arterial catheterization. In: Silverstein DC, Hopper K (eds). *Small Animal Critical Care Medicine*. Saunders-Elsevier, St. Louis, ch 49.

7 Hughes D, Beal MW (2000). Emergency vascular access. *Vet Clin North Am Small Anim Pract* 30(3):491–507.

8 Beal MW, Hughes D (2000). Vascular access: theory and techniques in the small animal emergency patient. *Clin Tech Small Anim Pract* 15(2):101–109.

9 Bliss SP, Bliss SK, Harvey KJ (2002). Use of recombinant tissue-plasminogen activator in a dog with chylothorax secondary to catheter-associated thrombosis of the cranial vena cava. *J Am Anim Hosp Assoc* 38:431–435.

10 Marsh-Ng ML, Burney DP, Garcia J
    (2007). Surveillance of infections
    associated with intravenous catheters in
    dogs and cats in an intensive care unit.
    J Am Anim Hosp Assoc **43**(1):13–20.
11 Lobetti RG, Joubert KE, Picard J, *et al.*
    (2002). Bacterial colonization of
    intravenous catheters in young dogs
    suspected to have parvoviral enteritis.
    J Am Vet Med Assoc **220**(9)1321–1324.
12 Coolman BR, Marretta SM, Kakoma I, *et
    al.* (1998). Cutaneous antimicrobial
    preparation prior to intravenous catheter
    preparation in healthy dogs: clinical
    microbiological, and histopathological
    evaluation. *Can Vet J* **39**(12):757–763.
13 Mathews KA, Brooks MJ, Valliant AE
    (1996). A prospective study of
    intravenous catheter contamination. *J Vet
    Emerg Crit Care* **6**(1):33–42.

CHAPTER 3

1 Rudloff E, Kirby R (1998). Fluid
   therapy: crystalloids and colloids. *Vet
   Clin North Am Small Anim Pract*
   28(2):297–328.
2 Rudloff E, Kirby R (2001). Colloid and
   crystalloid resuscitation. *Vet Clin North
   Am Small Anim Pract* **31**(6):1207–1229.
3 Griffel MI, Kaufman BS (1992).
   Pharmacology of colloids and
   crystalloids. *Crit Care Clinics*
   8(2):235–253.
4 Mathews KA (1998). The various types
   of parenteral fluids and their indications.
   Vet Clin North Am Small Anim Pract
   28(3):483–513.
5 DiBartola SP, Bateman S (2006).
   Introduction to fluid therapy. In:
   DiBartola SP (ed). *Fluid, Electrolyte, and
   Acid–Base Disorders*, 3rd edn. Saunders-
   Elsevier, St. Louis, pp. 325–344.
6 MacMillan KL (2003). Neurological
   complications following treatment of
   canine hypoadrenocorticism. *Can Vet J*
   44(6):490–492.
7 Rozanski E, Rondeau M (2002).
   Choosing fluids in traumatic

hypovolemic shock, the role of
crystalloids, colloids, and hypertonic
saline. *J Am Anim Hosp Assoc*
38:499–501.
8 Wingfield WE (2002). Fluid and
   electrolyte therapy. In: Wingfield WE,
   Raffe MR (eds). *The Veterinary ICU
   Book*. Teton NewMedia, Jackson,
   pp.166–188.
9 Starling EH (1894). On the absorption
   of fluids from the connective tissue
   spaces. *J Physiol* **140**:312–326.
10 Waddell LS, Brown AJ (2009).
    Hemodynamic monitoring. In:
    Silverstein DC, Hopper K (eds). *Small
    Animal Critical Care Medicine.*
    Saunders-Elsevier, St Louis,
    pp. 859–864.
11 Rudloff E, Kirby R (2000). Colloid
    osmometry. *Clin Tech Small Anim Pract*
    15(3):119–125.
12 Gabel JC, Scott RL, Adair TH, *et al.*
    (1980). Errors in calculated oncotic
    pressure in the dog. *Am J Physiol*
    239(Heart Circ Physiol **8**):H810–H812.
13 Navar PD, Navar LG (1977).
    Relationship between colloid osmotic
    pressure and plasma protein
    concentration in the dog. *Am J Physiol*
    233(2):H295–H298.
14 Brown A, Dusza K, Boehmer J (1994).
    Comparison of measured and calculated
    values for colloid osmotic pressure in
    hospitalized animals. *Am J Vet Res*
    55(7):910–915.
15 Machon RG, Raffe MR, Robinson EP
    (1995). Central venous pressure
    measurements in the caudal vena cava of
    sedated cats. *J Vet Emerg Crit Care*
    5(2):121–129.
16 Berg RA, Lloyd TR, Donnerstein RL
    (1992). Accuracy of central venous
    pressure monitoring in the
    intraabdominal inferior vena cava: a
    canine study. *J Pediatr* **120**(1):67–71.
17 Syring RS, Otto CM, Drobatz KJ
    (2001). Hyperglycemia in dogs and cats
    with head trauma:122 cases
    (1997–1999). *J Am Vet Med Assoc*
    218(7):1124–1129.

CHAPTER 4

1 Mathews KA (1998). Various types of parenteral fluids and their indications. *Vet Clin North Am Small Anim Pract* 28(3):483-513, 1998.
2 Rudloff E, Kirby R (1998). Crystalloids and colloids. *Vet Clin North Am Small Anim Pract* 28(2):297–328.
3 Moore L (1998). Fluid therapy in the hypoproteinemic patient. *Vet Clin North Am Small Anim Pract* 28(3):709–715.
4 Bumpus SE, Haskins SC, Kass PH (1998). Effect of synthetic colloids on refractometric readings of total solids. *J Vet Emerg Crit Care* 8(1):21–26.
5 Kirby R, Rudloff E (1997). The critical need for colloids: maintaining fluid balance. *Comp Cont Educ Pract Vet* 19(6):705–717.
6 Rudloff E, Kirby R (2000). Colloid osmometry. *Clin Tech Small Anim Pract* 15(3):119–125.
7 Rackow EC, Falk JL, Fein IA (1983). Fluid resuscitation in circulatory shock: a comparison of the cardiorespiratory effects of albumin, hetastarch, and saline solutions in patients with hypovolemic and septic shock. *Crit Care Med* 11(11):839–850.
8 Suda S (2000). Hemodynamic and pulmonary effects of fluid resuscitation from hemorrhagic shock in the presence of mild pulmonary edema. *Masui* 49(12):1339–1348.
9 Gabel JC, Scott RL, Adair TH, *et al.* (1980). Errors in calculated oncotic pressure in the dog. *Am J Physiol* 239(Heart Circ Physiol 8):H810–H812.
10 Navar PD, Navar LG (1977). Relationship between colloid osmotic pressure and plasma protein concentration in the dog. *Am J Physiol* 233(2):H295–H298.
11 Brown A, Dusza K, Boehmer J (1994). Comparison of measured and calculated values for colloid osmotic pressure in hospitalized animals. *Am J Vet Res* 55(7):910–915.
12 Griffel MI, Kaufman BS (1992). Pharmacology of colloids and crystalloids. *Crit Care Clinics* 8(2):235–253.
13 Smiley LE (1992). The use of hetastarch for plasma expansion. *Prob Vet Med* 4(4):652–667.
14 Yacobi A, Gibson TP, McEntegart CM, Hulse JD (1982). Pharmacokinetics of high molecular weight hydroxyethyl starch in dogs. *Res Commun Chem Pathol Pharmacol* 36:199–204.
15 Thompson WL, Fukushima T, Rutherford RC, Walton RP (1970). Intravascular persistence, tissue storage and excretion of hydroxyethyl starch. *Surg Gynecol Obstet* 131:965–972.
16 Madjdpour C, Thyes C, Buclin T, *et al.* (2007). Novel starches: single dose pharmacokinetics and effects on blood coagulation. *Anesthesiology* 106(1):132–143.
17 Cheng C, Lerner MA, Lichenstein S, *et al.* (1966). Effect of hydroxyethyl starch on hemostasis. *Surgical Forum: Metabolism* 17:48–50.
18 Wierenga JR, Jandrey KE, Haskins SC, Tablin F (2007). *In vitro* comparison of the effects of two forms of hydroxyethyl starch solutions on platelet function in dogs. *Am J Vet Res* 68(6):605–609.
19 Thyes C, Madjdpour C, Frascarolo P, *et al.* (2006). Effect of high- and low-molecular weight low-substituted hydroxyethyl starch on blood coagulation during acute normovolemic hemodilution in pigs. *Anesthesiology* 105(6):1228–1237.
20 Mailloux L, Swartz CD, Cappizzi R, *et al.* (1967). Acute renal failure after administration of low-molecular weight dextran. *N Engl J Med* 277:1113.
21 Modig J (1988). Beneficial effects of dextran 70 versus Ringer's acetate on pulmonary function, hemodynamics and survival in porcine endotoxin shock model. *Resuscitation* 16:1-12.
22 Drobatz KJ, Macintire DK (1996). Heat-induced illness in dogs: 42 cases

(1976–1993). *J Am Vet Med Assoc* **209**(11):1894–1899.

23 Grimes JA, Schmiedt CW, Cornell KK, Radlinsky MAG (2011). Identification of risk factors for septic peritonitis and failure to survive following gastrointestinal surgery in dogs. *J Am Vet Med Assoc* **234**(4):486–494.

24 Mazzaferro EM, Rudloff E, Kirby R (2002). Role of albumin replacement in the critically ill veterinary patient. *J Vet Emerg Crit Care* **12**(2):113–124.

25 Mathews KA (2008). The therapeutic use of 25% human serum albumin in critically ill dogs and cats. *Vet Clin North Am Small Anim Pract* **38**(3):595–605.

26 Trow AV, Rozanski EA, deLaforcade AM, Chan DL (2008). Evaluation of use of human albumin in critically ill dogs: 73 cases (2003–2006). *J Am Vet Med Assoc* **233**(4):607–612.

27 Hughes D, Boag AK (2006). Fluid therapy with macromolectular plasma volume expanders. In: DiBartola SP (ed). *Fluid, Electrolytes, and Acid–Base Disorders in Small Animal Practice.* Saunders-Elsevier, St. Louis, pp. 621–634.

28 Cohn LA, Kerl ME, Lenox CE, Livingston RS, Dodham JR (2007). Response of healthy dogs to infusions of human serum albumin. *Am J Vet Res* **68**(6):657–663.

29 Martin LG, Luther TY, Alperin DA, Gay JM, Hines SA (2008). Serum antibodies against human albumin in critically ill and healthy dogs. *J Am Vet Med Assoc* **232**(7):1004–1009.

30 Francis AH, Martin LG, Haldorson GJ, *et al.* (2007). Adverse reactions suggestive of type III hypersensitivity in six healthy dogs given human albumin. *J Am Vet Med Assoc* **230**(6):873–879.

CHAPTER 5

1 Lower R (1989). A Treatise on the Heart on the Movement and Colour of the Blood and on the Passage of the Chyle into the Blood. In: Frankin KJ (ed). Special edition, The Classics of Medicine Library, Gryphi Editions, Birmingham, p. xvi.

2 Giger U (2009). Transfusion medicine. In: Silverstein DC, Hopper K (eds). *Small Animal Critical Care Medicine.* Saunders-Elsevier, St. Louis, ch 66, pp. 281–286.

3 Hohenhaus AE (2006). Blood transfusion and blood substitutes. In: DiBartola SP (ed). *Fluid, Electrolyte, and Acid–Base Disorders.* Saunders-Elsevier, St. Louis, pp. 567–583.

4 Wardrop KJ, Reine N, Birkenheuer A, *et al.* (2005). Canine and feline blood donor screening for infectious disease. ACVIM Consensus Statement. *J Vet Intern Med* **19**:135–142.

5 Giger U, Oakley D, Owens SD, Schantz F (2002). *Leishmania donovani* transmission by packed RBC transfusion to anemic dogs in the United States. *Transfusion* **42**(30):381–383.

6 Owens SD, Oakley DA, Marryott K, *et al.* (2001). Transmission of visceral leishmaniasis through blood transfusions from infected Foxhounds to anemic dogs. *J Am Vet Med Assoc* **219**(8):1076–1083.

7 Steiger K, Palos H, Giger U (2005). Comparison of various blood-typing methods for the feline AB blood group system. *Am J Vet Res* **66**(8):1393–1399.

8 Giger U, Stieger K, Palos H (2005). Comparison of various canine blood-typing methods. *Am J Vet Res* **66**(8):1386–1392.

9 Blais MC, Berman L, Oakley DA, Giger U (2007). Canine *Dal* blood type: a red cell antigen lacking in some Dalmatians. *J Vet Intern Med* **21**:281–286.

10 Giger U, Akol KG (1990). Acute hemolytic transfusion reaction in an Abyssinian cat with blood type B. *J Vet Intern Med* **4**(6):315–316.

11 Weinstein NM, Blais MC, Harris K, Oakley DA, Aronson LR, Giger U (2007). A newly recognized blood group in Domestic Shorthair cats: the Mik red cell antigen. *J Vet Intern Med* **21**:287–292.

12 Wardrop KJ (2007). New red blood cell antigens in dogs and cats: a welcome discovery. *J Vet Intern Med* **21**:205–206.

13 Giger U, Bucheler J (1991). Transfusion of type-A and type-B blood to cats. *J Am Vet Med Assoc* **198**(3):411–418.

14 Bucheler J, Giger U (1990). Transfusion of type A and B blood in cats. *J Vet Intern Med* **4**(2):111.

15 Giger U, Gorman NT, Hubler M, *et al.* (1993). Frequencies of feline A and B blood types in Europe. *Anim Genet* **23**(Supp 1):17–18.

16 Giger U, Griot-Wenk M, Bucheler J, *et al.* (1991). Geographical variation of feline blood type frequencies in the United States. *Fel Pract* **19**:22–27.

17 Knottenbelt CM (2002). The feline AB blood group system and its importance in transfusion medicine. *J Fel Med Surg* **4**:69–76.

18 Auer L, Bell K (1981). The AB blood group system in cats. *Anim Blood Groups Biochem Genet* **12**:287–297.

19 Griot-Wenk ME, Callan MB, Casal ML, *et al.* (1996). Blood type AB in the feline AB blood group system. *Am J Vet Res* **57**:1438–1442.

20 Chiaramonte D (2004). Blood-component therapy: selection, administration and monitoring. *Clin Tech Small Anim Pract* **19**(2):63–67.

21 Jutkowitz LA (2004). Blood transfusion in the perioperative period. *Clin Tech Small Anim Pract* **19**(2):75–82.

20 Chiaramonte D (2004). Blood-component therapy: selection, administration and monitoring. *Clin Tech Small Anim Pract* **19**(2):63–67.

22 Weingart C, Giger U, Kohn B (2004). Whole blood transfusions in 91 cats: a clinical evaluation. *J Fel Med Surg* **6**(3):139–148.

23 Giger U, Gelens CJ, Callan MB, Oakley DA (1995). An acute hemolytic transfusion reaction caused by dog erythrocyte antigen 1.1 compatibility in a previously sensitized dog. *J Am Vet Med Assoc* **206**(9):1358–1362.

24 Haldane S, Roberts J, Marks SL, Raffe MR (2004). Transfusion medicine. *Comp Cont Educ Pract Vet* **26**(7):502–517.

25 Waddell LS, Holt DE, Hughes D, Giger U (2001). The effect of storage on ammonia concentration in canine packed red blood cells. *J Vet Emerg Crit Care* **11**(1):23–26.

26 Sprague WS, Hackett TB, Johnson JS, Swardson-Olver CJ (2003). Hemochromatosis secondary to repeated blood transfusions in a dog. *Vet Pathol* **40**(3):334–337.

CHAPTER 6

1 Rose BD (1994). Hyperosmolar states – hypernatremia. In: *Clinical Physiology of Acid–Base and Electrolyte Disorders*, 4th edn. McGraw-Hill.

2 Marks SL, Taboada J (1998). Hypernatremia and hypertonic syndromes. *Vet Clin North Am Small Anim Pract* **29**:533–543.

3 Manning AM (2001). Electrolyte disorders. *Vet Clin North Am Small Anim Pract* **31**(6):1289–1321.

4 Burkitt JM (2008). Sodium disorders. In: Silverstein DC, Hopper K (eds). *Small Animal Critical Care Medicine*. Elsevier Saunders, St. Louis, pp. 224–229.

5 Phillips SL, Polzin DJ (1998). Clinical disorders of potassium homeostasis. *Vet Clin North Am Sm Anim Pract* **28**(3):545–564.

6 Dow SW, LeCouteur RA, Fettman MJ, Spurgeon TL (1987). Potassium depletion in cats: hypokalemic polymopathy. *J Am Vet Med Assoc* **191**(12):1563–1568.

7 Dhupa N, Proulx J (1998). Hypocalcemia and hypomagnesemia. *Vet Clin North Am Small Anim Pract* **28**(3):587–608.

8 Martin LG, Matteson VL, Wingfield WE, *et al.* (1994). Abnormalities of serum magnesium in critically ill dogs: incidence and implications. *J Vet Emerg Crit Care* **4**:15.

9 Martin LG (1998). Hypercalcemia and hypermagnesemia. *Vet Clin North Am Small Anim Pract* **28**(3):565–585.

CHAPTER 7

1 Remillard RL, Darden DE, Michel KE, Marks SL, Buffington CA, Bunnell PR (2001). An investigation of the relationship between caloric intake and outcome in hospitalized dogs. *Vet Ther* **2**(4):301–310.

2 Lippert AC, Armstrong PJ (1989). Parenteral nutritional support. In: Kirk RW, Bonagura JD (eds). *Current Veterinary Therapy X*, pp. 25–30.

3 Lippert AC, Fulton RB, Parr AM (1993). A retrospective study of the use of total parenteral nutrition in dogs and cats. *J Vet Intern Med* **7**:52–64.

4 Remillard RL (2002). Nutritional support in critical care patients. *Vet Clin Small Anim Pract* **32**:1145–1164.

5 Reuter JD, Marks SL, Rogers QR, Farver TB (1998). Use of total parenteral nutrition in dogs: 209 cases (1988–1995). *J Vet Emerg Crit Care* **8**:201–213.

6 Remillard RL, Armstrong PJ, Davenport DJ (2000). Assisted feeding in hospitalized patients: enteral and parenteral nutrition. In: Hand MS, Thatcher CD, Remillard RL, Roudebush P (eds). *Small Animal Clinical Nutrition*, 4th edn. Mark Morris Institute, Walsworth, Marceline.

7 Chandler ML, Guilford WG, Payne-James J (2000). Use of peripheral parenteral nutritional support in dogs and cats. *J Am Vet Med Assoc* **216**(5):669–673.

8 Armstrong PJ, Lippert AC (1988). Selected aspects of enteral and parenteral nutritional support. *Semin Vet Med Surg (Small Anim)* **3**(3):216–226.

9 Freeman LM, Labato MA, Rush JE, Murtaugh RJ (1995). Nutritional support in pancreatitis: a retrospective study. *J Vet Emerg Crit Care* **5**(1):32–41.

10 Pyle SC, Marks SL, Kass PH (2004). Evaluation of complications and prognostic factors associated with administration of total parenteral nutrition in cats: 75 cases (1994–2001). *J Am Vet Med Assoc* **225**(2):242–250.

11 Mauldin GE, Reynolds AJ, Mauldin GN, Kallfelz FA (2001). Nitrogen balance in clinically normal dogs receiving parenteral nutrition solutions. *Am J Vet Res* **62**:912–920.

12 Walton RS, Wingfield WE, Ogilvie GK, *et al.* (1996). Energy expenditure in 104 postoperative and traumatically injured dogs with indirect calorimetry. *J Vet Emerg Crit Care* **6**:71–79.

13 O'Toole E, Miller CW, Wilson BA, Mathews KA, Davis C, Sears W (2004). Comparison of the standard predictive equation for calculation of resting energy expenditure with indirect calorimetry in hospitalized and healthy dogs. *J Am Vet Med Assoc* **225**(1):58–64.

14 Chan DL, Freeman LM, Rozanski EA, Rush JE (2001). Colloid osmotic pressure of parenteral nutrition components and intravenous fluids. *J Vet Emerg Crit Care* **11**(4):269–273.

15 Mathews KA (1998). The various types of parenteral fluids and their indications. *Vet Clin Small Anim Pract* **28**(3):483–513.

16 Lewis LD, Morris ML, Hand MS (1990). *Small Animal Clinical Nutrition*. Mark Morris Associates, Topeka, pp.5-35–5-41.

17 Chan DL, Freeman LM, Labato MA, Rush JE (2002). Retrospective evaluation of partial parenteral nutrition in dogs and cats. *J Vet Intern Med* **16**:440–445.

18 Mohr AJ, Leisewitz AL, Jacobson LS, Steiner JM, Ruaux CG, Williams DA (2003). Effect of early enteral nutrition on intestinal permeability, intestinal protein loss, and outcome in dogs with severe parvoviral enteritis. *J Vet Intern Med* **17**(6):791–798.

CHAPTER 8

1 Day TK, Bateman S (2006). Shock syndromes. In: DiBartola SP (ed). *Fluid, Electrolyte, and Acid–Base Disorders in Small Animal Practice*. Saunders-Elsevier, St. Louis, ch 23, pp. 540–564.

2 Pachtinger GE, Drobatz K (2008). Assessment and treatment of hypovolemic states. *Vet Clin North Am Small Anim Pract* **38**:629–643.

3 Rudloff E, Kirby R (2008). Fluid resuscitation and the trauma patient. *Vet Clin North Am Small Anim Pract* **38**:645–652.

4 Rudloff E, Kirby R (2001). Colloid and crystalloid resuscitation. *Vet Clin North Am Small Anim Pract* **31**(6): 1207–1229.

5 de Papp E, Drobatz KJ, Hughes D (1999). Plasma lactate concentration as a predictor of gastric necrosis and survival among dogs with gastric dilatation-volvulus: 102 cases (1995–1998). *J Am Vet Med Assoc* **215**(1):49–52.

6 Zacher LA, Berg J, Shaw SP, Kudei RK (2010). Association between outcome and changes in plasma lactate concentration during presurgical treatment in dogs with gastric dilatation-volvulus: 64 cases (2002–2008). *J Am Vet Med Assoc* **236**(8):892–897.

7 Lagutchik MS, Ogilvie GK, Hackett TB, et al. (1998). Increased lactate concentrations in ill and injured dogs. *J Vet Emerg Crit Care* **8**:117–126.

8 Boag AK, Hughes D (2005). Assessment and treatment of perfusion abnormalities in the emergency patient. *Vet Clin North Am Small Anim Pract* **35**:319–342.

9 Moore KE, Murtaugh RJ (2001). Pathophysiologic characteristics of hypovolemic shock. *Vet Clin North Am Small Anim Pract* **31**(6):1115–1128.

10 Rozanski E, Rondeau M (2002). Choosing fluids in traumatic hypovolemic shock: the role of crystalloids, colloids and hypertonic saline. *J Am Anim Hosp Assoc* **38**(6):499–501.

11 Mandell DC, King LG (1998). Fluid therapy in shock. *Vet Clin North Am Small Anim Pract* **28**(3):623–645.

12 Stump DC, Strauss RG, Hennksen RA, et al. (1985). Effect of hydroxyethyl starch on blood coagulation, particularly factor VIII. *Transfusion* **25**:349.

13 Schertel ER, Schneider DA, Zissimos AG (1985). Cardiopulmonary reflexes induced by osmolality changes in the airways and pulmonary vasculature. *Fed Proc* **44**:835.

14 Brown AJ, Mandell DC (2009). Cardiogenic shock. In: Silverstein DC, Hopper K (eds). *Small Animal Critical Care Medicine*. Saunders-Elsevier, St. Louis, ch 35, pp. 146–150.

15 Mittleman Boller E, Otto CM (2009). Ch 107: Septic shock. In: Silverstein DC, Hopper K (eds). *Small Animal Critical Care Medicine*. Saunders-Elsevier, St. Louis, ch 107, pp. 459–463.

16 Brady CA, Otto CM, Van Winkel TJ, King LG (2000). Severe sepsis in cats: 29 cases (1986–1998). *J Am Vet Med Assoc* **217**(40):531–535.

17 Purvis D, Kirby R (1994). Systemic inflammatory response syndrome: septic shock. *Vet Clin North Am Small Anim Pract* **24**:1225.

18 Smarick SD, Haskins SC, Aldrich J, et al. (2004). Incidence of catheter-associated urinary tract infections among dogs in a small animal intensive care unit. *J Am Vet Med Assoc* **224**(12):1936–1940.

CHAPTER 9

1 Mohr AJ, Leisewitz AL, Jacobson LS, Steiner JM, Ruaux CG, Williams DA (2003). Effect of early enteral nutrition on intestinal permeability, intestinal protein loss, and outcome in dogs with severe parvoviral enteritis. *J Vet Intern Med* **17**(6):791–798.

Index